Pocket Atlas
of Pulse Diagnosis

Zheng-Hong Lin

Doctor of Chinese Medicine
Taipei, Taiwan

154 illustrations

Thieme
Stuttgart · New York

Library of Congress Cataloging-in-Publication Data is available from the publisher.

This book is an authorized and revised translation of the 1st Chinese edition published and copyrighted 2004 in Taiwan by Big Forest Publishing Co., Ltd. Title of the Chinese edition: 脈診: 一學就通

Translator: Mei Li, New York, US

Important note: Medicine is an ever-changing science undergoing continual development. Research and clinical experience are continually expanding our knowledge, in particular our knowledge of proper treatment and drug therapy. Insofar as this book mentions any dosage or application, readers may rest assured that the authors, editors, and publishers have made every effort to ensure that such references are in accordance with **the state of knowledge at the time of production of the book.**

Nevertheless, this does not involve, imply, or express any guarantee or responsibility on the part of the publishers in respect to any dosage instructions and forms of applications stated in the book. **Every user is requested to examine carefully** the manufacturers' leaflets accompanying each drug and to check, if necessary in consultation with a physician or specialist, whether the dosage schedules mentioned therein or the contraindications stated by the manufacturers differ from the statements made in the present book. Such examination is particularly important with drugs that are either rarely used or have been newly released on the market. Every dosage schedule or every form of application used is entirely at the user's own risk and responsibility. The authors and publishers request every user to report to the publishers any discrepancies or inaccuracies noticed. If errors in this work are found after publication, errata will be posted at www.thieme.com on the product description page.

© 2008 Georg Thieme Verlag,
Rüdigerstrasse 14, 70469 Stuttgart, Germany
http://www.thieme.de
Thieme New York, 333 Seventh Avenue,
New York, NY 10001, USA
http://www.thieme.com

Cover design: Thieme Publishing Group
Typesetting by Druckerei Sommer,
Feuchtwangen
Printed in Germany by APPL, aprinta druck,
Wemding, Germany

ISBN TPS: 978-3-13-144051-8
ISBN TPN: 978-1-58890-623-6

1 2 3 4 5 6

Preface

Palpation is an extremely important component of Chinese medical diagnosis. The four diagnostic methods comprise the combination of "Inspection, Listening and Smelling, Inquiry, and Palpation." According to many years of experience, I have found in clinical diagnosis that palpation can be likened to having the effects of "adding the final touches that bring a work of art to life" (*huà lóng diǎn jīng*, 畫龍點睛) and "heading straight for the goal" (*lín mén yì jiǎo,* 臨門一腳). In other words, if one can use "palpation" to confirm what one has deduced from inspection, listening and smelling, and inquiry, one can avoid making erroneous diagnoses as well as increase diagnostic accuracy.

The idea that the pulse alone enables the practitioner to arrive at an accurate diagnosis is a misconception. Throughout history, however, scholars have misled people into believing that some physicians possessed such miraculous abilities as to be able to feel a patient's pulse and divulge everything about the person's illness, without having to go through the other three methods of examination (i.e., inspection, listening and smelling, and inquiry). This is, indeed, a misunderstanding of Chinese medicine.

Objectively speaking, in certain classical disease patterns, for instance, in liver blood deficiency patients, the left bar (*guān*, 關) position of the pulse will be either soggy (*rú*, 濡) or vacuous (*xū*, 虛). In this situation, one can certainly acquire some useful knowledge from the pulse palpation; however, this does not mean that there is liver blood deficiency whenever one encounters a soggy or vacuous pulse in the left bar position.

This is because, in disease patterns, there is a differentiation between true, false, vacuity, and repletion. In regard to the relationship between disease patterns and pulse manifestation, there are two types: mutual agreement between the pattern and the pulse, and mutual contradiction between the pattern and the pulse. Because a person's constitution varies from individual to individual, and the disease condition also differs from person to person, would it not seem too subjective and risky to a responsible doctor with a rational approach to rely solely on palpation as a means of flaunting his or her medical skill, as opposed to objectively utilizing all four pillars—inspection, listening and smelling, inquiry, and palpation—in disease diagnosis?

For instance, the famous physician, Wáng Shū-Hé (王叔和) of the late *Hàn* (漢) dynasty, said, in *The Pulse Canon* (*Mài Jīng*, 脈經):

"Those who go on to study medicine, due to ignorance and lack of clarity about the pulse, in addition to prejudices and biases that exist amongst themselves, in order to flaunt their ability, will mistakenly diagnose mild diseases as more severe ones, to the point where they sever their chance of survival (by ruining their own reputation); there definitely is a reason for this."

Wáng Shū-Hé furthermore stated:

"If the sunken pulse (*chén mài*, 沉脈) is diagnosed as the hidden pulse (*fú mài*, 伏脈), the treatment would be erroneous; if the moderate pulse (*huǎn mài*, 緩脈) is diagnosed as the slow pulse (*chí mài*, 遲脈), a dangerous consequence would immediately follow. Furthermore, one type of disease pattern can often possess several different pulse manifestations, while different diseases can, indeed, have identical pulse manifestations. With that said, how can one not be meticulous and careful?

"Therefore, in ancient times, even if a doctor is as wise and highly-skilled as Biǎn Què (扁鵲), careful consideration is still required during diagnosis. Although Zhāng Zhòng-Jǐng (張仲景) excelled at pattern differentiation, he still would carefully examine the disease pattern; if he found any areas he was unclear or uncertain about, he would thoroughly analyze the details to gain more insight."

The above illustrates, precisely, a rational approach.

If palpation is seen as the highest realm of Chinese medical diagnosis, this is an overexaggeration of its role and results in the casting aside of the other three diagnostic methods (inspection, listening and smelling, and inquiry). It is as ridiculous as wanting to paint a dragon, but painting only the eyes without the body.

This book portrays the shapes of the 28 pulses in detail, cites commonly encountered clinical disease patterns, and extracts text from Volume 8 of *The Pulse Canon* to further explain the application of palpation in diagnosis. In short, the knowledge contained within this book allows the beginner to establish a proper foundation in the study of pulse diagnosis, at the same time re-emphasizing the fact that no matter how important palpation is in diagnosis, it still cannot replace Chinese medical diagnosis as a whole.

Zheng-Hong Lin

■ Table of Contents

3 Analyses of the Pulse Manifestations and Signs of Common Diseases 93

4 *The Pulse Canon* (*Mài Jīng*, 脈經), Volume 8, written by Wáng Shū-Hé, Imperial Physician of the *Jin* (晉) Dynasty 173

1 The Origin and Development of Pulse Diagnosis

■ The Forerunner of the Pulse Theory: Qín Yuè Rén (秦越人), a.k.a. Biǎn Què (扁鵲)

So far, there is still insufficient evidence regarding exactly when pulse diagnosis originated; however, according to relevant records of historical data, the earliest time period that pulse diagnosis can be traced back to is before the 6th century BCE.

Qín Yuè Rén (6th century BCE) was a renowned physician during the Warring States period (475–221 BCE) and was known to the world as Biǎn Què.

Biǎn Què was well known because of his special skills in pulse diagnosis, for which Sī-Mǎ Qiān (司馬遷) praised him in *Historical Records* (*Shǐ Jì*, 史記): "Anything that is said about the pulse starts with Biǎn Què." From this, we can deduce that as early as the 6th century BCE, Biǎn Què was already utilizing the method of pulse examination to diagnose disease.

■ The Prophet of the Pulse Theory: Yī Huǎn (醫緩)

Yī Huǎn lived during the Spring Autumn Period in the State of *Qín* (秦). According to *Left Transmission* (*Zuǒ Chuán*, 左傳), Qín Huán Gōng (秦桓公, 603–577 BCE) sent Yī Huǎn to the State of *Jìn* (晉) to treat a monarch by the name of Jǐng Gōng (景公). During the diagnosis, he spoke bluntly without any inhibitions, saying that the disease was untreatable. This was because the disease condition had already reached the end-stage severity of being "above the *huāng* (肓) and below the *gāo* (膏)." (See Glossary for definitions.) Even if the disease were treated with *biān* (砭) stone therapy, acupuncture, and moxibustion, it would be of no use; even if it were treated with medicinals, the medicinals would not reach the location of the disease. The patient had absolutely no chance of survival. This is also where the saying "the disease has attacked the vitals; a disease that is beyond cure (*bìng rù gāo huāng*, 病入膏肓)" originates from.

How did Yī Huǎn know to diagnose this as a disease of the *gāo huāng* (within the viscera and bowels)? Did he only rely on the three examinations (inspection, listening and smelling, and inquiry) to arrive at such a bold conclusion?

From this, we can deduce that Yī Huǎn certainly incorporated the reference of the pulse diagnostic method into his diagnosis for him to dare risk his life by uttering such a definitive, yet dangerous, statement in front of Jǐng Gōng.

Without a doubt, this also explains the contributory role of the pulse in diagnosis.

■ The Earliest Ancestors of the Pulse Theory: *Method of Pulse Examination* (Mài Fǎ, 脈法) and *Fatal Symptoms of the Yin and Yang Vessels* (Yīn Yáng Mài Sǐ Hòu, 陰陽脈死候)

In early 1973 to 1974, the *Hàn* Dynasty *Mǎ Wáng Duī* (馬王堆) Tomb Number 3 was unearthed in Changsha City, the modern capital of Hunan Province; this contained the following 11 medical texts:

- *Moxibustion Classic of the Eleven Vessels of the Legs and Arms* (Zú Bì Shí Yī Mài Jiǔ Jīng, 足臂十一脈灸經)
- *Moxibustion Classic on the Eleven Yin and Yang Vessels* (Yīn Yáng Shí Yī Mài Jiǔ Jīng, 陰陽十一脈灸經), *Volumes 1 and 2*
- *Method of Pulse Examination* (Mài Fǎ, 脈法)
- *Fatal Symptoms of the Yin and Yang Vessels* (Yīn Yáng Mài Sǐ Hòu, 陰陽脈死候)
- *Formulas for Fifty-two Diseases* (Wǔ Shí Èr Bìng Fāng, 五十二病方)
- *Abstinence from Grains and Consumption of Qi* (Què Gǔ Shí Qì, 卻穀食氣)
- *Illustrations of Conduction Exercise* (Dǎo Yǐn Tú, 導引圖)
- *Formulas for Life Preservation* (Yǎng Shēng Fāng, 養生方)
- *Formulas for Miscellaneous Cures* (Zá Liáo Fāng, 雜療方)
- *Book on Childbirth* (Tāi Chǎn Shū, 胎產書)

According to certain evidence, the time period in which these books were written was no later than the transition between the *Qín* and *Hàn* dynasties (late 3rd century BCE) and no earlier than *The Yellow Emperor's Inner Canon*.

Of these 11 books, *Moxibustion Classic of the Eleven Vessels of the Legs and Arms* (Zú Bì Shí Yī Mài Jiǔ Jīng, 足臂十一脈灸經) and *Moxibustion Classic on the Eleven Yin and Yang Vessels* (Yīn Yáng Shí Yī Mài Jiǔ Jīng, 陰陽十一脈灸經), Volumes 1 and 2, give a comprehensive description of the pathways of 11 channel vessels, their direction of flow, and their disease indications. These are, by far, the earliest texts related to channel theory.

The *Method of Pulse Examination* (Mài Fǎ, 脈法) and *Fatal Symptoms of the Yin and Yang Vessels* (Yīn Yáng Mài Sǐ Hòu, 陰陽脈死候) include records of simple descriptions of pulse manifestation and diagnosis, and are perhaps earlier versions of *The Yellow Emperor's Inner Canon* (Huáng Dì Nèi Jīng, 黃帝內經).

■ The Cornerstone of the Pulse Theory: *The Yellow Emperor's Inner Canon* (Huáng Dì Nèi Jīng, 黃帝內經)

The Yellow Emperor's Inner Canon consists of two parts—*The Magic Pivot* (Líng Shū, 靈樞) and *Plain Questions* (Sù Wèn, 素問)—each volume containing 81 chapters with a total of more than 80 000 characters.

The period in which *The Yellow Emperor's Inner Canon* was written has not yet been determined; however, it should not be later than the Warring States period. From the content, we can tell that it was not written by one person during one era; rather, it is possible it was written by many doctors throughout history who borrowed the names of the Yellow Emperor and his officials, Qí Bó (岐伯), Léi Gōng (雷公), Guǐ Yú Qū (鬼臾區), Bó Gāo (伯高), and others.

The Yellow Emperor's Inner Canon was probably derived from the fundamental theories of *Method of Pulse Examination* (Mài Fǎ, 脈法) and *Fatal Symptoms of the Yin and Yang Vessels* (Yīn Yáng Mài Sǐ Hòu, 陰陽脈死候). In *Plain Questions*, *Treatise on the Three Positions and Nine Indicators* (Sù Wèn, Sān Bù Jiǔ Hòu Lùn, 素問,三部九候論), the pulse diagnostic method of the three positions and nine indicators was first established.

Detailed explanations of the clinical applications of pulse theory and pulse manifestation can be found in:
- *Plain Questions*, *Treatise on the Essential Subtleties of the Pulse* (Sù Wèn, Mài Yào Jīng Wēi Lùn, 素問, 脈要精微論)
- *Plain Questions*, *Qi and Manifestations of Healthy Persons* (Sù Wèn, Píng Rén Qì Xiàng Lùn, 素問,平人氣象論)
- *Plain Questions*, *The Jade Swivel Treatise on True Visceral Pulses* (Sù Wèn, Yù Jī Zhēn Zàng Lùn, 玉機真臟論)

- *Plain Questions, Treatise on the Three Positions and Nine Indicators* (Sù Wèn, Sān Bù Jiǔ Hòu Lùn, 素問, 三部九候論)
- *Plain Questions, A Separate Treatise on the Channel Vessels* (Sù Wèn, Jīng Mài Bié Lùn, 素問, 經脈別論)
- *Plain Questions, General Treatise on Vacuity and Repletion* (Sù Wèn, Tōng Píng Xū Shí Lùn, 通評虛實論)
- *Plain Questions, Treatise on Major Strange Diseases* (Sù Wèn, Dà Qí Lùn, 大奇論).

■ The Revolutionary Text on the Pulse Theory: *The Classic of Difficult Issues* (Nàn Jīng, 難經)

The Classic of Difficult Issues was written later than *The Yellow Emperor's Inner Canon*. Tradition has it that Biǎn Què wrote this text. However, conclusions from the research of later generations confirmed that other doctors of the past supplemented and contributed to the writing of this book with their collective revisions, so this text was not created by one person during one era.

The Classic of Difficult Issues, which is based on *The Yellow Emperor's Inner Canon*, elaborates on the essence of the *Plain Questions* and *The Magic Pivot* in a question-and-answer format. The whole book is divided into 81 difficult issues, of which the first and the 22nd are discussions on pulse manifestation.

The main distinguishing feature of *The Classic of Difficult Issues* is its mention of a brand new thesis regarding the "Three Positions and Nine Indicators" model. For instance, *The Classic of Difficult Issues* assigns the viscera and bowels to different pulse positions according to their exterior–interior relationships; for example, the large intestine belongs to the right inch (*cùn*, 寸) position, the small intestine belongs to the left inch position, and the hand reverting *yin* pericardium network vessel and hand lesser *yang* triple burner channel belong to the right cubit (*chǐ*, 尺) position. This thesis is nothing like that of *The Yellow Emperor's Inner Canon*; because of this difference, doctors of later generations held varying opinions on the pulse positions of the viscera and bowels as put forth by the "Three Positions and Nine Indicators" model.

■ The Implementers of the Pulse Theory:
On Cold Damage and Miscellaneous Diseases (Shāng Hán Zá Bìng Lùn, 傷寒雜病論)

On Cold Damage and Miscellaneous Diseases was written in the late *Hàn* dynasty (206 BCE–220 CE) by Zhāng Zhòng-Jǐng (張仲景), who lived from 150 to 219 CE.

On Cold Damage and Miscellaneous Diseases inherited the basic theories of *The Yellow Emperor's Inner Canon* and *The Classic of Difficult Issues*. It applied the pulse diagnostic method to clinical diagnosis and established the principle of "treatment according to pattern differentiation (*biàn zhèng lùn zhì*, 辨證論治)." Two chapters in this book (*Píng Mài Fǎ* [平脈法] and *Biàn Mài Fǎ* [辨脈法]) discuss the clinical applications of the pulse theory in detail.

In *On Cold Damage and Miscellaneous Diseases*, for the diagnosis and treatment of miscellaneous diseases from external contraction and internal damage, the principles of the prescription and usage of herbal medicinals are based on the transmutation of pulse manifestation. This book, except for one third of the content that comprises records of the pulse theory, divides the pulse manifestation into two categories (*yin* and *yang*) in order to diagnose the advancement, regression, and progression of disease. As *On Cold Damage* states, "The large, floating, rapid, stirred, and slippery pulses are *yang*; the sunken, rough, weak, stringlike, and faint pulses are *yin*." It also states, "A *yang* pulse seen in a *yin* disease means that the patient will live; a *yin* pulse seen in a *yang* disease means that the patient will die."

■ The Unifier of the Pulse Theory:
The Pulse Canon (Mài Jīng, 脈經)

The Pulse Canon was written by Wáng Shū-Hé (王叔和, 201–280 CE) some time during the period from the end of the *Hàn* dynasty (206 BCE–220 CE) to the Western *Jìn* Dynasty (265–316 CE). It is the first monograph on pulse theory in the history of Chinese medicine.

The Pulse Canon firmly established the names of the 24 types of pulse manifestations.

fú	浮	kōu	芤
hóng	洪	huá	滑
shuò	數	cù	促
xián	弦	jǐn	緊
chén	沉	fú	伏
gé	革	shí	實
wēi	微	sè	澀
xì	細	ruǎn	軟
ruò	弱	xū	虛
sàn	散	huǎn	緩
chí	遲	jié	結
dài	代	dòng	動

In addition, it described the shape of each pulse and how to differentiate between similar pulses.

Aside from the soft pulse (ruǎn mài, 軟脈), which was later renamed the soggy pulse (rú mài, 濡脈), and the four new additions (the long, short, firm, and racing pulses), the 24 types of pulse mentioned in *The Pulse Canon* were adopted and utilized by later generations of doctors up to the present day.

■ The Composer of the Pulse Theory: *Pulse Rhymes* (Mài Jué, 脈訣)

Pulse Rhymes was written by Gāo Yáng-Shēng (高陽生), who lived during the Six Dynasties period (222–589 CE). It is the first medical text to expound and elaborate on pulse theory through rhymed verses.

Pulse Rhymes has over 200 rhymed verses. Because the written language of the content is easy to understand, recite, and memorize, this text has remained extremely popular among beginners, and has contributed to the dissemination of the study of the pulse throughout the generations.

■ The Critic of the Pulse Theory:
Corrections of Pulse Rhymes
(Mài Jué Kān Wù, 脈訣刊誤)

Corrections of Pulse Rhymes was written by Dài Qǐ-Zōng (戴啟宗) in the *Yuán* (元) dynasty (1279–1368 CE). It is the first critique on the pulse theory. Since there were some incomplete theses in *Pulse Rhymes*, many doctors raised their differing views on these various subjects in written form, of which *Corrections of Pulse Rhymes* was the most detailed.

Corrections of Pulse Rhymes is based on the theories of *The Yellow Emperor's Inner Canon*, *The Classic of Difficult Issues*, Zhāng Zhòng-Jǐng, and Wáng Shū-Hé. It is also directed at the shortcomings of *Pulse Rhymes*, and introduced new theses on the descriptions and indications of the pulse shape.

■ The Summarizer of the Pulse Theory:
The Lakeside Master's Study of the Pulse
(Bīn Hú Mài Xué, 瀕湖脈學)*

The Lakeside Master's Study of the Pulse was written by Lǐ Shí Zhēn (李時珍) in the *Míng* (明) dynasty (1368–1644 CE). It is a continuation of the fundamental theories set forth in *The Pulse Canon*, and a summary of the collective experience of previous generations who lived before the *Míng* Dynasty. The contents are divided into two main sections: *Four Syllable Rhymes* (Sì Yán Jué, 四言訣) and *Seven Syllable Rhymes* (Qī Yán Jué, 七言訣).

Four Syllable Rhymes is considered to be a brief introduction to the book. The content includes the physiology of the channel vessels, the mechanism of the formation of the pulse manifestation, the method of pulse examination, the features of all the pulses, the indications of the individual pulses, and the pulse manifestations of various diseases.

Seven Syllable Rhymes is the section containing commentary, in which the features and indications of each of the 27 pulses are described separately. It also discusses how to differentiate between similar pulses.

Lǐ Shí Zhēn (*Collection of Ancient and Modern Books: Category of Medicine, Complete Collection, No. 77 – Method of Pulse Examination, Pulse Rhymes*) emphasized the correlation of all four examinations and opposed the concept of re-

---

* a.k.a. "*Bīn Hú Sphymology*" (Wiseman/Feng)

lying solely on pulse examination in the determination of disease conditions. He categorized 24 pulses into seven exterior pulses, eight interior pulses, and nine principle pulses. The floating, large, rapid, stirred, and slippery pulses were considered *yang* pulses, while the sunken, short, rough, weak, and faint pulses were considered *yin* pulses.

The **seven exterior pulses** (*qī biǎo mài*, 七表脈) are floating (*fú*, 浮), scallion-stalk (*kōu*, 芤), slippery (*huá*, 滑), replete (*shí*, 實), stringlike (*xián*, 弦), tight (*jǐn*, 緊), and surging (*hóng*, 洪).

The **eight interior pulses** (*bā lǐ mài*, 八裡脈) are faint (*wēi*, 微), sunken (*chén*, 沉), moderate (*huǎn*, 緩), rough (*sè*, 濇 [=澀]), slow (*chí*, 遲), hidden (*fú*, 伏), soggy (*rú*, 濡), and weak (*ruò*, 弱).

The **nine principle pulses** (*jiǔ dào mài*, 九道脈) are long (*cháng*, 長), short (*duǎn*, 短), vacuous (*xū*, 虛), skipping (*cù*, 促), bound (*jié*, 結), intermittent (*dài*, 代), firm (*láo*, 牢), stirred (*dòng*, 動), and fine (*xì*, 細).

2 Differentiation of the Twenty-eight Pulses

▪ Palpation

Chinese medical diagnosis comprises four examinations: inspection, listening and smelling, inquiry, and palpation. Here, palpation refers to pulse diagnosis, also known as pulse examination. Palpation, at its earliest stage of development, was the "ubiquitous palpation method" (*biàn zhěn fǎ*, 遍诊法), namely, palpation of the arteries located in the head, hand, and foot regions; it was later narrowed down to what is presently known as palpation of the wrist pulse, located at the part of the wrist through which the radial arteries and the lung channel pass. From palpation of the wrist pulse, one can determine whether the pathological changes belong to the exterior or interior, cold or hot, and vacuity or repletion patterns.

Principles of Pulse Manifestation

The heart governs the blood and vessels: The heart propels the blood in the blood vessels; this produces a pulsation in the vessels, forming the pulse beat. It must be noted that the movement of the blood in the vessels requires not only the beating of the heart, but also the cooperation of the lung, spleen, liver, and kidney.

The lung faces the hundred vessels: The blood vessels of the whole body assemble in the lung. The lung governs *qi*; blood cannot be distributed throughout the entire body until it is disseminated by lung *qi*.

The spleen governs control of the blood: In order for blood to circulate within the vessels without spilling out of them, it relies on the controlling function of spleen *qi*.

The liver governs storage of the blood: The liver regulates the *qi* dynamic so that it is smooth and unimpeded. It also regulates the volume of blood in the body.

The kidney governs storage of essence: Essence can be transformed into *qi*, and is the root of the *yang qi* of the body. Furthermore, essence can also be transformed into blood, since it is one of the substances that give rise to blood production.

Therefore, the formation of pulse manifestation is intimately related to the *qi* and blood of the viscera (*zàng*, 臟) and bowels (*fŭ*, 腑).

Identification of Disease Using Pulse Diagnosis

The formation of the pulse manifestation is related to the changes in the *qi* and blood of the viscera and bowels; when a person is sick, the movement of the blood in the vessels will inevitably be affected, producing a change in the pulse manifestation. Although pathological changes can be extremely complex, one can still differentiate (from detectable changes in the pulse manifestation) the location of the disease, the characteristic of the disease, and the exuberance and debilitation of right (*zhèng*, 正) and evil (*xié*, 邪).

▓ The General Rules of Pulse Diagnosis

A floating pulse (*fú mài*, 浮脈) usually denotes an exterior pattern, while a sunken pulse (*chén mài*, 沉脈) usually indicates an interior pattern.

A slow (*chí mài*, 遲脈) pulse generally points to cold, whereas a rapid (*shuò*, 數) pulse usually indicates heat.

If palpation reveals a vacuous, forceless pulse, this generally indicates a vacuity pattern. If it reveals a replete, forceful pulse, this usually indicates a repletion pattern.

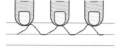

Floating level
Middle level
Deep level

Inch (*cùn*, 寸)   Bar (*guān*, 关)   Cubit (*chǐ*, 尺)

Floating pulse: generally indicates an exterior pattern.

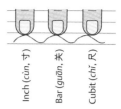

Inch (*cùn*, 寸)   Bar (*guān*, 关)   Cubit (*chǐ*, 尺)

Sunken pulse: generally indicates an interior pattern.

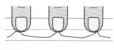

Floating level
Middle level
Deep level

Inch (*cùn*, 寸)   Bar (*guān*, 关)   Cubit (*chǐ*, 尺)

Slow pulse: generally indicates a cold pattern.

Inch (*cùn*, 寸)   Bar (*guān*, 关)   Cubit (*chǐ*, 尺)

Rapid pulse: generally indicates a heat pattern.

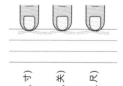

Floating level
Middle level
Deep level

Inch (*cùn*, 寸)   Bar (*guān*, 关)   Cubit (*chǐ*, 尺)

Vacuous pulse: generally indicates a vacuity pattern.

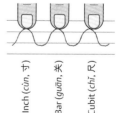

Inch (*cùn*, 寸)   Bar (*guān*, 关)   Cubit (*chǐ*, 尺)

Replete pulse: generally indicates a repletion pattern.

■ Positions of the Pulse

Diagnostic Method of the Wrist Pulse

The wrist pulse is divided into three sections: inch (*cùn*, 寸), bar (*guān*, 關), and cubit (*chǐ*, 尺). The bony prominence proximal to the wrist (styloid process of the radius) is the bar, in front of the bar is the inch, and behind the bar is the cubit. The wrist pulse of each hand is divided into these three sections, making a total of six pulse positions.

Each of the three pulse positions can also be divided into three depths for pulse examination: superficial, middle, and deep. This system of pulse examination is known as the "Three Positions and Nine Indicators" (*sān bù jiǔ hòu*, 三部九候).

Visceral *Qi* Associated with the Wrist Pulse

Skilled doctors of the past held differing views regarding the reflections of visceral *qi* in wrist pulse diagnosis. Generally, the inch, bar, and cubit of the right hand can be divided to reflect the lung, spleen, and kidney (Life Gate [*mìng mén*, 命門]); and the inch, bar, and cubit of the left hand can be divided to reflect the heart, liver, and kidney, respectively.

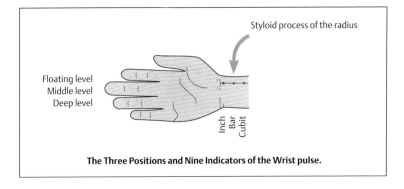

The Three Positions and Nine Indicators of the Wrist pulse.

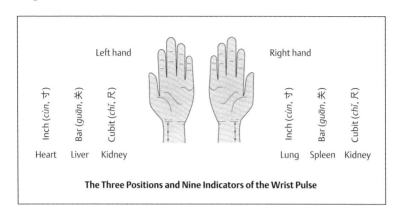

The Three Positions and Nine Indicators of the Wrist Pulse

Cautions of Using Palpation in Diagnosis

Before undertaking a pulse examination, the practitioner must allow the patient to rest, to maintain a state of calmness, and to avoid any interference from the external environment. This allows the patient's qi and blood to remain tranquil. When the practitioner is feeling the pulse, the patient's arm should be placed at the same height as that of the heart. The palm should be flat and facing upward, allowing the blood to flow smoothly. The practitioner should first locate the bar (*guān*, 关) pulse position by pressing the middle finger on the bony prominence (styloid process of the radius). The inch (*cùn*, 寸) position is located with the index finger, and the cubit (*chǐ*, 尺) position is located with the ring finger.

After accurately locating the pulse positions, the three fingers should be curved, to resemble the shape of a bow, so that the fingers are evenly lined up and the finger pads are pressing on the pulse. Three different finger strengths (light, medium, and heavy) can be exerted to feel the pulse at the three different depths in order to determine the pulse manifestation. This is known as "lifting, pressing, and searching." Using light finger pressure to press on the skin is called "lifting," also known as feeling the pulse at the superficial level, or feeling the pulse with light pressure. Using heavy finger pressure to press on the sinews and bones is called "pressing," also known as feeling the pulse at the deep level, or feeling the pulse with heavy pressure. Using neither light nor heavy pressure to shift and change the amount of strength exerted while attentively feeling for the pulse is known as "searching."

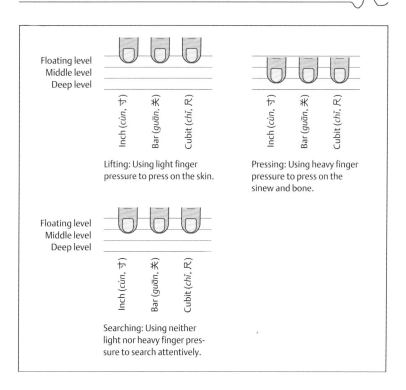

Floating level
Middle level
Deep level

Inch (*cùn*, 寸) Bar (*guān*, 关) Cubit (*chǐ*, 尺)

Lifting: Using light finger pressure to press on the skin.

Inch (*cùn*, 寸) Bar (*guān*, 关) Cubit (*chǐ*, 尺)

Pressing: Using heavy finger pressure to press on the sinew and bone.

Floating level
Middle level
Deep level

Inch (*cùn*, 寸) Bar (*guān*, 关) Cubit (*chǐ*, 尺)

Searching: Using neither light nor heavy finger pressure to search attentively.

Rate of Pulse Manifestation

When feeling the pulse, the practitioner's breathing should be even and steady, using the duration of one inhalation and one exhalation to calculate the patient's pulse rate.

One inhalation and exhalation is one respiration. Normally, a person's pulse will beat twice during one inhalation, and twice during one exhalation. Between inhalation and exhalation, there is one beat. Altogether, a normal pulse beats four to five times per respiration (on average, there being 17–18 respirations per minute, equal to 72–80 beats per minute).

When taking the pulse, the general requirement is to feel the pulse for 50 beats. This mainly serves to diagnose whether or not the pulse is skipping (*cù*, 促), bound (*jié*, 结), or intermittent (*dài*, 代).

However, during clinical pulse examination, depending on specific circumstances, one can adjust the length of pulse examination.

The Normal Pulse Manifestation

The normal pulse manifestation must possess the following three characteristics: the presence of stomach (*qi*), spirit, and root.

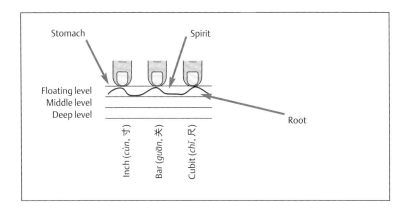

◼ Presence of Stomach (*qi*)

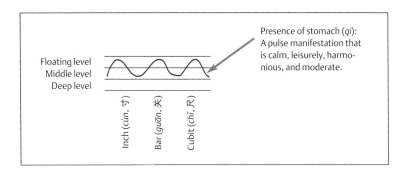

Presence of stomach (*qi*): A pulse manifestation that is calm, leisurely, harmonious, and moderate.

The stomach is the origin of the body's *qi* and blood of acquired constitution. Thus, the presence of stomach *qi* indicates that the pulse manifestation has force and spirit, and the absence of stomach *qi* then represents lack of force and spirit in the pulse.

The normal pulse manifestation is neither floating nor sunken, and neither fast nor slow. It is calm and leisurely, as well as harmonious and moderate. This is known as presence of stomach *qi*.

When illness occurs, regardless of whether the pulse is floating, sunken, slow, or rapid, it can, as long as it is both harmonious and moderate, still be considered a pulse that possesses stomach *qi*.

▓ Presence of Spirit

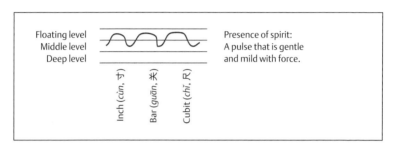

Floating level
Middle level
Deep level

Inch (*cùn*, 寸)   Bar (*guān*, 关)   Cubit (*chǐ*, 尺)

Presence of spirit:
A pulse that is gentle
and mild with force.

The heart governs the blood and stores the spirit. When *qi* and blood are abundant, the pulse manifestation naturally has spirit. A pulse that has spirit is gentle and mild, has force, and has consistency of rhythm.

When illness occurs, even if there is a pathological pulse that is stringlike (*xián*, 弦), the pulses are all known as having presence of spirit as long as there is a gentle and mild quality within the stringlike quality, or there is a pathological pulse that is slightly weak but has within that slight weakness slowness without complete lack of force.

▓ Presence of Root

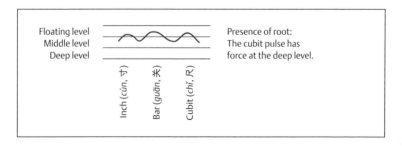

Floating level
Middle level
Deep level

Inch (*cùn*, 寸)   Bar (*guān*, 关)   Cubit (*chǐ*, 尺)

Presence of root:
The cubit pulse has
force at the deep level.

The kidney is the root of congenital constitution. When kidney *qi* is sufficient, the pulse will naturally have root. When taking the pulse, the state of the kidney can be perceived through the cubit (*chǐ*, 尺) position. Feeling the pulse at the deep level can also reveal the health of the kidney.

If the pulse has force at all three positions (inch, bar, and cubit) when palpated at the deep level, or as long as the cubit pulse has force when palpated at the deep level, it is still considered a pulse that has root.

Therefore, when a person falls ill, if there is still kidney *qi* left, the kidney *qi* can be felt through the cubit pulse, indicating that the basis of congenital constitution has not yet expired and that the patient still has a chance to recover.

Other Particular Aspects of the Pulse

Seasons: Due to climatic influences, the normal pulse can adapt and change according to the corresponding seasons. In the spring the pulse is stringlike, in the summer it is surging, in the autumn it is floating, and in the winter it is sunken.

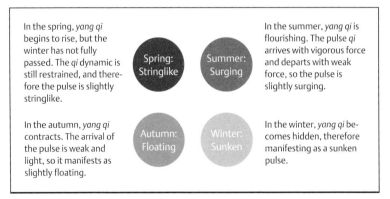

In the spring, *yang qi* begins to rise, but the winter has not fully passed. The *qi* dynamic is still restrained, and therefore the pulse is slightly stringlike.

Spring: Stringlike

Summer: Surging

In the summer, *yang qi* is flourishing. The pulse *qi* arrives with vigorous force and departs with weak force, so the pulse is slightly surging.

In the autumn, *yang qi* contracts. The arrival of the pulse is weak and light, so it manifests as slightly floating.

Autumn: Floating

Winter: Sunken

In the winter, *yang qi* becomes hidden, therefore manifesting as a sunken pulse.

Gender: The pulse of a female is usually slightly faster than that of a male. A pregnant woman will usually exhibit a gentle pulse that is slippery and rapid.
Age: The younger the age, the faster the pulse. An infant's pulse is 120–140 beats per minute, whereas that of a 5–6-year-old child is 90–110 beats per minute.

Body type: People of tall stature will usually have longer pulses, and those of short stature will usually have shorter pulses. Skinny people have thin flesh, so their pulses tend to be floating. The adipose layers of fat people are thick, so that their pulses are usually more sunken than normal.

The anomalous pulses: Although the six pulses manifest in some people as deep and fine, they are not considered pathological. These are known as the "six *yin* pulses." In others, the six pulses manifest as surging and large, yet there is also no pathology. These are known as the "six *yang* pulses."

There are still others whose pulses are rather peculiar. For example, if the pulse cannot be felt at the wrist, but instead appears in the area that stretches from the cubit position to the back of the hand, this is known as the "oblique running pulse" (*xié fēi mài*, 斜飛脈). Similarly, if the pulse is found on the dorsal aspect of the wrist, this is called the "pulse on the back of the wrist" (*fǎn guān mài*, 反關脈), also known as the "dorsal styloid pulse."

In short, none of the abnormal pulse locations mentioned above are considered pathological.

■   The Guiding Principles of Pulse Manifestation

There are a total of 28 different pulses. When learning the pulses, they can be divided into the following six categories: floating, sunken, slow, rapid, vacuous, and replete. Studying the 28 pulses in detail after first grasping these six categories of pulse will make it easier to remember them.

1. **The Category of the Floating Pulse (*Fú Mài*, 浮脈):** Consists of floating, surging, soggy, scattered, scallion-stalk, and drumskin pulses, which are all located at the superficial level.
2. **The Category of the Sunken Pulse (*Chén Mài*, 沉脈):** Consists of sunken, hidden, confined, and weak pulses, which are all located at the deep level.
3. **The Category of the Slow Pulse (*Chí Mài*, 迟脈):** Consists of slow, moderate, rough, and bound pulses, which are all slow.
4. **The Category of the Rapid Pulse (*Shuò Mài*, 數脈):** Consists of rapid, racing, skipping, and stirred pulses, which are all fast.
5. **The Category of the Vacuous Pulse (*Xū Mài*, 虛脈):** Consists of vacuous, faint, fine, intermittent, and short pulses, which are all forceless.
6. **The Category of the Replete Pulse (*Shí Mài*, 實脈):** Consists of replete, long, slippery, stringlike, and tight pulses, which are all forceful.

The Category of the Floating Pulse (*Fú Mài,* 浮脉)

Consists of floating, surging, soggy, scattered, scallion-stalk, and drum-skin pulses, which are all located at the superficial level.

The characteristic of the floating pulses: The pulse is located at the surface of the skin (with the exception of the surging pulse).

In other words, as long as the finger presses lightly on the skin, the beating of the pulse can be felt. If heavy pressure is applied, the pulse will then feel weak or hollow.

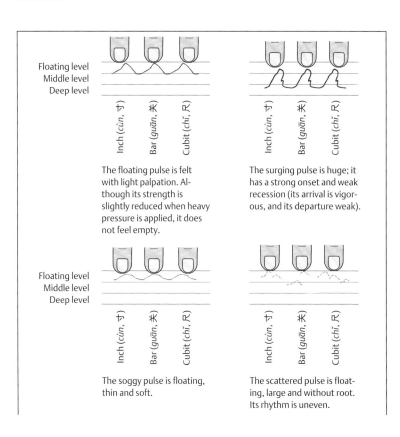

The floating pulse is felt with light palpation. Although its strength is slightly reduced when heavy pressure is applied, it does not feel empty.

The surging pulse is huge; it has a strong onset and weak recession (its arrival is vigorous, and its departure weak).

The soggy pulse is floating, thin and soft.

The scattered pulse is floating, large and without root. Its rhythm is uneven.

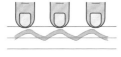

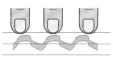

Floating level
Middle level
Deep level

Inch (cùn, 寸)   Bar (guān, 关)   Cubit (chǐ, 尺)

Inch (cùn, 寸)   Bar (guān, 关)   Cubit (chǐ, 尺)

The scallion-stalk pulse is floating, large, and empty in the middle level; it feels like the stalk of a scallion.

The drumskin pulse is stringlike, urgent, and empty in the middle level. It feels like the surface of a drum.

The Category of the Sunken Pulse (*Chén Mài*, 沉脉)

Consists of sunken, hidden, confined, and weak pulses, which are all located at the deep level.

The characteristic of the sunken pulses: The pulse is located at the depth of the sinews and bones.

In other words, when the fingers press lightly on the skin, the beating of the pulse is not very prominent. Heavy pressure must be applied to reach the depth of the sinews and bones in order to feel the beating of the pulse.

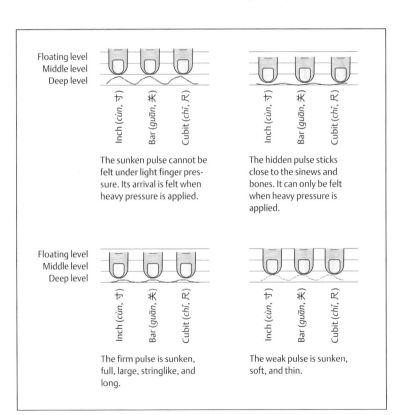

The sunken pulse cannot be felt under light finger pressure. Its arrival is felt when heavy pressure is applied.

The hidden pulse sticks close to the sinews and bones. It can only be felt when heavy pressure is applied.

The firm pulse is sunken, full, large, stringlike, and long.

The weak pulse is sunken, soft, and thin.

The Category of the Slow Pulse (*Chí Mài,* 遲脈)

Consists of slow, moderate, rough, and bound pulses, which are all slow.

The characteristic of the slow pulses: The frequency of the pulse beat is slow, causing a reduction in the pulse rate.

As for the depth, the pulse can be felt at all three levels (superficial, middle, and deep).

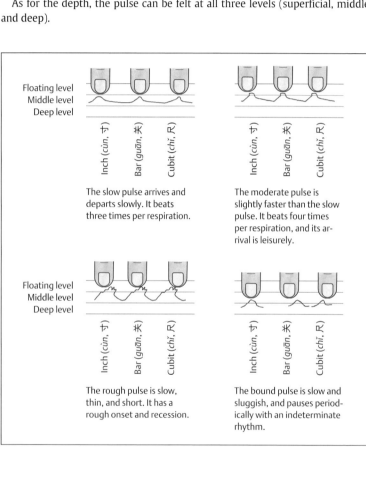

The slow pulse arrives and departs slowly. It beats three times per respiration.

The moderate pulse is slightly faster than the slow pulse. It beats four times per respiration, and its arrival is leisurely.

The rough pulse is slow, thin, and short. It has a rough onset and recession.

The bound pulse is slow and sluggish, and pauses periodically with an indeterminate rhythm.

The Category of the Rapid Pulse (*Shuò Mài*, 數脈)

Consists of rapid, racing, skipping, and stirred pulses, which are all fast.

The characteristic of the rapid pulses: The frequency of the pulse is fast, therefore causing the rate of the pulse to be excessively high.

This type of pulse can be palpated at all three levels (superficial, middle, and deep).

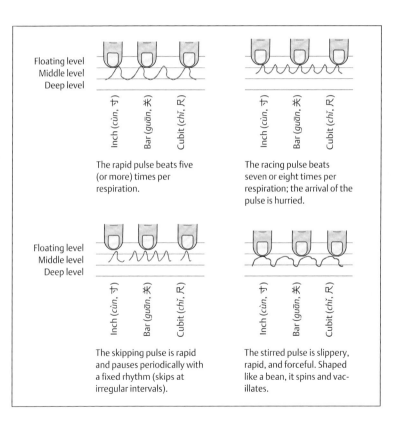

The rapid pulse beats five (or more) times per respiration.

The racing pulse beats seven or eight times per respiration; the arrival of the pulse is hurried.

The skipping pulse is rapid and pauses periodically with a fixed rhythm (skips at irregular intervals).

The stirred pulse is slippery, rapid, and forceful. Shaped like a bean, it spins and vacillates.

The Category of the Vacuous Pulse (*Xū Mài*, 虚脉)

Consists of vacuous, faint, fine, intermittent, and short pulses, which are all forceless.

The characteristic of the vacuous pulses: The pulse is soft and forceless.

The scope of the vacuous pulse category is wide. Regardless of the depth or frequency, as long as the beating of the pulse is weak and the quality of the pulse is soft, it belongs to the vacuous pulse category.

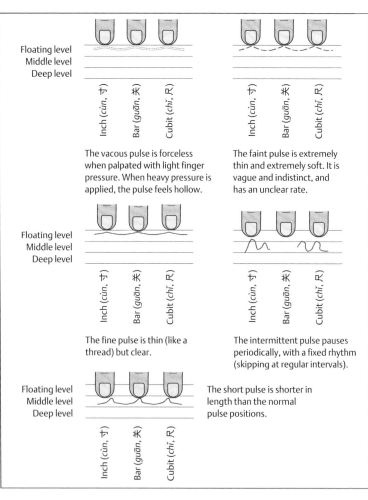

The vacous pulse is forceless when palpated with light finger pressure. When heavy pressure is applied, the pulse feels hollow.

The faint pulse is extremely thin and extremely soft. It is vague and indistinct, and has an unclear rate.

The fine pulse is thin (like a thread) but clear.

The intermittent pulse pauses periodically, with a fixed rhythm (skipping at regular intervals).

The short pulse is shorter in length than the normal pulse positions.

The Category of the Replete Pulse (*Shí Mài*, 實脈)

Consists of replete, long, slippery, stringlike, and tight pulses, which are all forceful.

The characteristic of the replete pulses: The pulse is strong and forceful.

The scope of the replete pulse category is wide. Regardless of the depth or frequency, as long as the beating of the pulse is strong and the quality of the pulse is large, it belongs to the replete pulse category.

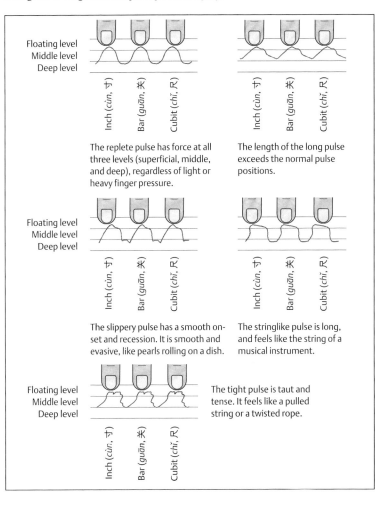

The replete pulse has force at all three levels (superficial, middle, and deep), regardless of light or heavy finger pressure.

The length of the long pulse exceeds the normal pulse positions.

The slippery pulse has a smooth onset and recession. It is smooth and evasive, like pearls rolling on a dish.

The stringlike pulse is long, and feels like the string of a musical instrument.

The tight pulse is taut and tense. It feels like a pulled string or a twisted rope.

The Characteristics and Indications of the Twenty-eight Pulses

One	Indications of the Floating Pulse Category	Characteristics
1	The **floating pulse** indicates an exterior pattern (the pulse must be floating and forceful). It is also seen in wind–water (*fēng shuǐ*, 風水).	The floating pulse is felt with light palpation. Although its strength is slightly reduced when heavy pressure is applied, it does not feel empty.
2	The **surging pulse** indicates a heat pattern.	The surging pulse is huge; it has a strong onset and weak recession (vigorous arrival and weak departure).
3	The **soggy pulse** indicates vacuity of *yin*, *yang*, *qi*, and blood.	The soggy pulse is floating, thin and soft.
4	The **scattered pulse** indicates dispersal of original *qi*.	The scattered pulse is floating, large, and without root. Its rhythm is uneven.
5	The **scallion-stalk pulse** indicates blood loss or damaged *yin*.	The scallion-stalk pulse is floating, large, and hollow; it feels like the stalk of a scallion.
6	The **drumskin pulse** indicates blood collapse or seminal loss.	The drumskin pulse is stringlike, urgent, and empty in the middle level. It feels like the surface of a drum.
Two	Indications of the Sunken Pulse Category	Characteristics
7	The **sunken pulse** indicates an interior pattern. A sunken, forceful pulse points to interior repletion; a sunken, forceless pulse points to interior vacuity.	The sunken pulse cannot be felt with light finger pressure. Its arrival is felt only when heavy pressure is applied.

Two	Indications of the Floating Pulse Category	Characteristics
8	The **hidden pulse** indicates evil block (*xié bì*, 邪閉), reversal pattern (*jué zhèng*, 厥證), or pain.	The hidden pulse sticks close to the sinews and bones. It can only be felt when heavy pressure is applied.
9	The **firm pulse** indicates exuberant internal *yin* cold.	The firm pulse is sunken, replete, large, stringlike, and long.
10	The **weak pulse** indicates *qi* and blood depletion.	The weak pulse is sunken, soft, and thin.
Three	Indications of the Slow Pulse Category	Characteristics
11	The **slow pulse** indicates a cold pattern. A slow, forceful pulse indicates cold repletion (note: or repletion heat); a slow, forceless pulse indicates vacuity cold.	The slow pulse arrives and departs slowly. It beats three times per respiration.
12	The **moderate pulse** indicates dampness or spleen vacuity.	The moderate pulse is slightly faster than the slow pulse. It beats four times per respiration. Its arrival is leisurely.
13	The **rough pulse** indicates damaged essence, blood vacuity, *qi* stagnation, or blood stasis.	The rough pulse is slow, thin, and short. It has a harsh onset and recession.
14	The **bound pulse** indicates exuberance of *yin* humor and *qi* bind. It also indicates debilitation of *qi* and blood.	The bound pulse is slow and sluggish, and pauses periodically with an indeterminate rhythm (skips at irregular intervals).
Four	Indications of the Rapid Pulse Category	Characteristics
15	The **rapid pulse** indicates heat. The rapid pulse can also indicate a vacuity pattern.	The rapid pulse beats five or more times per respiration.

Four	Indications of the Rapid Pulse Category	Characteristics
16	The **racing pulse** indicates extreme *yang* and exhaustion of *yin*. It can also indicate impending desertion of original *qi*.	The racing pulse beats seven or eight times per respiration; the arrival of the pulse is hurried.
17	The **skipping pulse** indicates *yang* exuberance and repletion heat, blood stasis, phlegm–rheum, or stagnation of abiding food. It can also indicate debilitation of original *qi*.	The skipping pulse is rapid and pauses periodically with an indeterminate rhythm (skips at irregular intervals).
18	The **stirred pulse** indicates pain or fright.	The stirred pulse is slippery, rapid and forceful. Shaped like a bean, it spins and vacillates.
Five	Indications of the Vacuous Pulse Category	Characteristics
19	The **vacuous pulse** indicates a vacuity pattern.	The vacuous pulse is forceless when palpated with light finger pressure. When heavy pressure is applied, the pulse feels empty.
20	The **faint pulse** indicates *qi* and blood vacuity.	The faint pulse is extremely thin and extremely soft. It is vague and indistinct, and has an unclear rate.
21	The **fine pulse** indicates dual vacuity of *qi* and blood, all types of vacuity, or taxation detriment (*láo sǔn*, 劳损).	The fine pulse is thin (like a thread) yet clear.
22	The **intermittent pulse** indicates debilitation of visceral *qi*.	The intermittent pulse pauses periodically and has a fixed rhythm (skips at regular intervals).

Five	Indications of the Vacuous Pulse Category	Characteristics
23	The **short pulse** indicates *qi* disease. A short, forceless pulse indicates *qi* vacuity; a short, forceful pulse indicates *qi* repletion.	The short pulse is shorter in length than the normal pulse positions.

Six	Indications of the Rapid Pulse Category	Characteristics
24	The **replete pulse** indicates a repletion pattern. It is also seen in patterns of *yin* cold and reversal cold.	The replete pulse has force at all three levels (superficial, middle, and deep), regardless of light or heavy finger pressure.
25	The **long pulse** indicates a *yang* pattern, such as superabundance of liver *yang* or patterns of *yang* exuberance with internal heat.	The length of the long pulse exceeds the normal pulse positions.
26	The **slippery pulse** indicates phlegm–rheum, abiding food, repletion heat, or blood amassment (*xù xuè*, 蓄血).	The slippery pulse has a smooth onset and recession. It is smooth and evasive, like pearls rolling on a dish.
27	The **stringlike pulse** indicates liver and gallbladder disease, phlegm–rheum, all types of pain, or malaria. The stringlike pulse can also indicate vacuity.	The stringlike pulse is long, and feels like the string of a musical instrument.
28	The **tight pulse** indicates cold, pain, or abiding food (*sù shí*, 宿食).	The tight pulse is taut and tense. It feels like a pulled string or a twisted rope.

Classification of the Twenty-eight Pulses

The Category of the Floating Pulse (*Fú Mài*, 浮脈)

Consists of floating, surging, soggy, scattered, scallion-stalk, and drumskin pulses, which are all located at the superficial level.

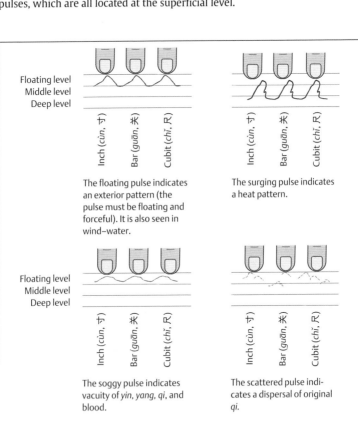

The floating pulse indicates an exterior pattern (the pulse must be floating and forceful). It is also seen in wind–water.

The surging pulse indicates a heat pattern.

The soggy pulse indicates vacuity of *yin, yang, qi,* and blood.

The scattered pulse indicates a dispersal of original *qi*.

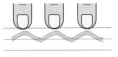

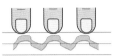

Floating level
Middle level
Deep level

Inch (cùn, 寸)
Bar (guān, 关)
Cubit (chǐ, 尺)

Inch (cùn, 寸)
Bar (guān, 关)
Cubit (chǐ, 尺)

The scallion-stalk pulse indicates blood loss or damaged *yin*.

The drumskin pulse indicates blood collapse or seminal loss.

The Category of the Sunken Pulse (*Chén Mài*, 沉脈)

Consists of sunken, hidden, confined, and weak pulses, which are all located at the deep level.

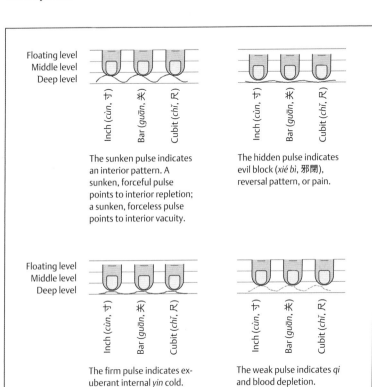

The sunken pulse indicates an interior pattern. A sunken, forceful pulse points to interior repletion; a sunken, forceless pulse points to interior vacuity.

The hidden pulse indicates evil block (*xié bì*, 邪閉), reversal pattern, or pain.

The firm pulse indicates exuberant internal *yin* cold.

The weak pulse indicates *qi* and blood depletion.

The Category of the Slow Pulse (*Chí Mài*, 遲脈)

Consists of slow, moderate, rough, and bound pulses, which are all slow.

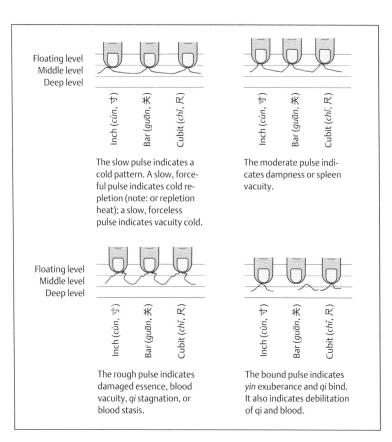

Floating level
Middle level
Deep level

Inch (*cùn*, 寸) Bar (*guān*, 夬) Cubit (*chǐ*, 尺)

The slow pulse indicates a cold pattern. A slow, forceful pulse indicates cold repletion (note: or repletion heat); a slow, forceless pulse indicates vacuity cold.

Floating level
Middle level
Deep level

Inch (*cùn*, 寸) Bar (*guān*, 夬) Cubit (*chǐ*, 尺)

The moderate pulse indicates dampness or spleen vacuity.

Floating level
Middle level
Deep level

Inch (*cùn*, 寸) Bar (*guān*, 夬) Cubit (*chǐ*, 尺)

The rough pulse indicates damaged essence, blood vacuity, *qi* stagnation, or blood stasis.

Floating level
Middle level
Deep level

Inch (*cùn*, 寸) Bar (*guān*, 夬) Cubit (*chǐ*, 尺)

The bound pulse indicates *yin* exuberance and *qi* bind. It also indicates debilitation of qi and blood.

The Category of the Rapid Pulse (*Shuò Mài*, 數脈)

Consists of rapid, racing, skipping, and stirred pulses, which are all fast.

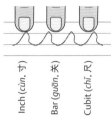

Floating level
Middle level
Deep level

Inch (*cùn*, 寸) Bar (*guān*, 关) Cubit (*chǐ*, 尺)

The rapid pulse indicates heat. The rapid pulse can also indicate a vacuity pattern.

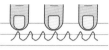

Inch (*cùn*, 寸) Bar (*guān*, 关) Cubit (*chǐ*, 尺)

The racing pulse indicates extreme *yang* and exhaustion of *yin*. It can also indicate impending original *qi* desertion.

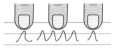

Floating level
Middle level
Deep level

Inch (*cùn*, 寸) Bar (*guān*, 关) Cubit (*chǐ*, 尺)

The skipping pulse indicates *yang* exuberance and repletion heat, blood stasis, phlegm–rheum, or stagnation of abiding food. It can also indicate debilitation of original *qi*.

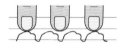

Inch (*cùn*, 寸) Bar (*guān*, 关) Cubit (*chǐ*, 尺)

The stirred pulse indicates pain or fright.

The Category of the Vacuous Pulse (*Xū Mài*, 虚脉)

Consists of vacuous, faint, fine, intermittent, and short pulses, which are all forceless.

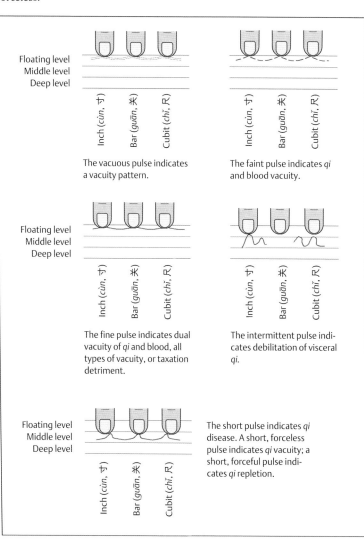

Floating level
Middle level
Deep level

Inch (*cùn*, 寸)   Bar (*guān*, 关)   Cubit (*chǐ*, 尺)

The vacuous pulse indicates a vacuity pattern.

Floating level
Middle level
Deep level

Inch (*cùn*, 寸)   Bar (*guān*, 关)   Cubit (*chǐ*, 尺)

The faint pulse indicates *qi* and blood vacuity.

Floating level
Middle level
Deep level

Inch (*cùn*, 寸)   Bar (*guān*, 关)   Cubit (*chǐ*, 尺)

The fine pulse indicates dual vacuity of *qi* and blood, all types of vacuity, or taxation detriment.

Floating level
Middle level
Deep level

Inch (*cùn*, 寸)   Bar (*guān*, 关)   Cubit (*chǐ*, 尺)

The intermittent pulse indicates debilitation of visceral *qi*.

Floating level
Middle level
Deep level

Inch (*cùn*, 寸)   Bar (*guān*, 关)   Cubit (*chǐ*, 尺)

The short pulse indicates *qi* disease. A short, forceless pulse indicates *qi* vacuity; a short, forceful pulse indicates *qi* repletion.

The Category of the Replete Pulse (*Shí Mài*, 實脈)

Consists of replete, long, slippery, stringlike, and tight pulses, which are all forceful.

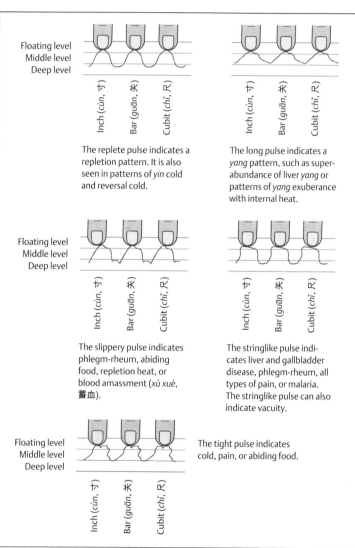

Floating level
Middle level
Deep level

Inch (*cùn*, 寸)   Bar (*guān*, 关)   Cubit (*chǐ*, 尺)

The replete pulse indicates a repletion pattern. It is also seen in patterns of *yin* cold and reversal cold.

The long pulse indicates a *yang* pattern, such as superabundance of liver *yang* or patterns of *yang* exuberance with internal heat.

Floating level
Middle level
Deep level

Inch (*cùn*, 寸)   Bar (*guān*, 关)   Cubit (*chǐ*, 尺)

The slippery pulse indicates phlegm-rheum, abiding food, repletion heat, or blood amassment (*xù xuè*, 蓄血).

The stringlike pulse indicates liver and gallbladder disease, phlegm-rheum, all types of pain, or malaria. The stringlike pulse can also indicate vacuity.

Floating level
Middle level
Deep level

Inch (*cùn*, 寸)   Bar (*guān*, 关)   Cubit (*chǐ*, 尺)

The tight pulse indicates cold, pain, or abiding food.

Differentiation of the Pulses and Their Corresponding Diseases

The Floating Pulse (*Fú Mài*, 浮脉)

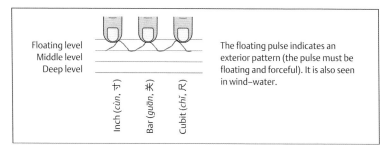

Floating level
Middle level
Deep level

Inch (*cùn*, 寸)
Bar (*guān*, 关)
Cubit (*chǐ*, 尺)

The floating pulse indicates an exterior pattern (the pulse must be floating and forceful). It is also seen in wind–water.

Pulse Manifestation

- The strength of the floating pulse is most prominent when palpated lightly. Although its strength is slightly reduced when heavy pressure is applied, it does not feel empty.
- The pulsation can be felt when the fingers press lightly on the surface of the skin. When heavier pressure is exerted, the pulsation under the fingers will be reduced. However, the pulse does not feel empty.

Pulse Principles

- When pathogenic *qi* invades the external aspect of the body through the fleshy exterior, there is a struggle between the defense *qi* of the body and the external evil. As a result, the vessel *qi* pulsates forcefully and the pulse is floating and clear (distinct).
- When the body is debilitated from enduring illness, the resulting internal depletion of *qi* and blood causes *yang qi* to float to the exterior because it is no longer able to attach itself to *yin* fluids. The pulse will then manifest as floating, large, and forceless.

Differentiation

The floating pulse is similar to the scallion-stalk, soggy, vacuous, and scattered pulses. The characteristic of these four pulse manifestations is that they are all located in the shallow part of the fleshy exterior; thus, they are easily confused with the floating pulse.

▦ Comparing the Pulses

- The shape of the floating pulse is neither large nor small. The strength of the floating pulse is most prominent under light palpation. Its strength is slightly reduced when heavy pressure is applied. However, the pulse does not feel empty.
- The location of the scallion-stalk pulse is at the superficial level. The shape of the pulse is large, yet it feels hollow. It feels like the stalk of a scallion.
- The location of the soggy pulse is at the superficial level. The shape of the pulse is thin and small, and its quality is soft.
- The vacuous pulse is weak and forceless, and its shape is thin and small. Furthermore, it feels empty.
- The scattered pulse is located at the superficial level. It feels as if it has no root. Its shape is thin and small, and its rhythm is uneven.

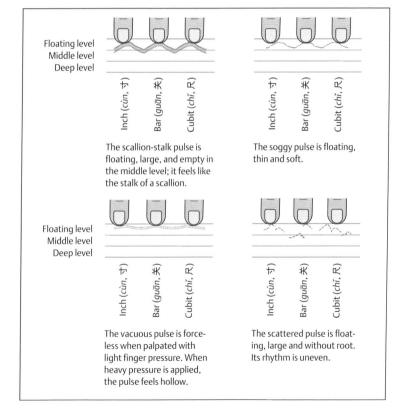

Floating level
Middle level
Deep level

Inch (cùn, 寸)   Bar (guān, 关)   Cubit (chǐ, 尺)

The scallion-stalk pulse is floating, large, and empty in the middle level; it feels like the stalk of a scallion.

Inch (cùn, 寸)   Bar (guān, 关)   Cubit (chǐ, 尺)

The soggy pulse is floating, thin and soft.

Floating level
Middle level
Deep level

Inch (cùn, 寸)   Bar (guān, 关)   Cubit (chǐ, 尺)

The vacuous pulse is forceless when palpated with light finger pressure. When heavy pressure is applied, the pulse feels hollow.

Inch (cùn, 寸)   Bar (guān, 关)   Cubit (chǐ, 尺)

The scattered pulse is floating, large and without root. Its rhythm is uneven.

■ Indications

- In general, when the floating pulse indicates an exterior pattern, it is usually forceful and neither large nor small.
- When the floating pulse indicates a vacuity pattern, it manifests as floating, large, and forceless.
- The floating pulse can also be felt in patients with wind–water (*fēng shuǐ*, 風水) or skin–water (*pí shuǐ*, 皮水). In other words, when wind evil mixes with water–damp and accumulates and obstructs the fleshy exterior, this can also give rise to a floating pulse.

■ Concurrent Pulses and their Indications

Concurrent Pulse Manifestations	Manifesting Symptoms
Floating and tight	Cold damage
Floating and moderate	Wind strike
Floating and rapid	Wind–heat
Floating and vacuous	Summerheat damage
Floating and surging	Exuberant heat
Floating and stringlike	Headache
Floating and slippery	Wind–phlegm

The Surging Pulse (*Hóng Mài*, 洪脈)

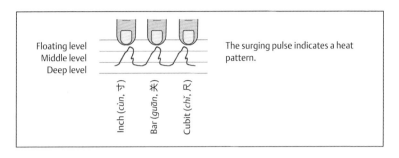

Floating level
Middle level
Deep level

Inch (*cùn*, 寸)
Bar (*guān*, 关)
Cubit (*chǐ*, 尺)

The surging pulse indicates a heat pattern.

▦ Pulse Manifestation

- The surging pulse is extremely large. It is shaped like a boat amidst the turbulence of great waves. It has a strong onset and weak recession.
- The surging pulse is floating and large. It is like a boat in turbulent waters. The force of the pulse is strong during the onset, after which it gradually diminishes. As a result, the departure of the pulse is milder in force and weaker in strength than its arrival.

▦ Pulse Principles

- Since evil heat can damage the *yin* fluids and lead to exuberance of *yang qi* assaulting the blood vessels, when evil heat blazes intensely within the body, the blood in the vessels is no match for the strength of the exuberant *yang qi*. As a result, the arteries expand, manifesting as the massive onset and weak recession that is characteristic of the surging pulse.

▦ Differentiation

The surging pulse is similar to the replete pulse. Both pulse manifestations are strong and forceful.

▦ Comparing the Pulses

- When pressed lightly, the surging pulse feels like a boat in turbulent waters: its onset is strong, and its recession weak. Its strength is diminished when palpated at the deep level.

- Although the replete pulse is not as unrestrained and vigorous, it is forceful when palpated with either light or heavy pressure. Both the onset and the recession of the pulse are extremely strong.

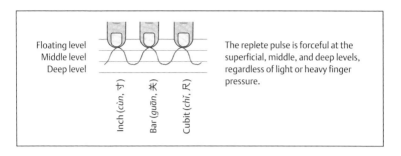

Floating level
Middle level
Deep level

Inch (*cùn*, 寸)
Bar (*guān*, 关)
Cubit (*chǐ*, 尺)

The replete pulse is forceful at the superficial, middle, and deep levels, regardless of light or heavy finger pressure.

▨ Indications

- The surging pulse indicates a heat pattern, usually due to extreme exuberance of *yang* heat, or to fire heat brewing internally. The symptoms produced include vexation and thirst, a red facial complexion, and generalized fever. As a result, the quality of the surging pulse is similar to a boat amidst turbulent waters, with a strong onset and weak recession.

The Soggy Pulse (*Rú Mài*, 濡脈)

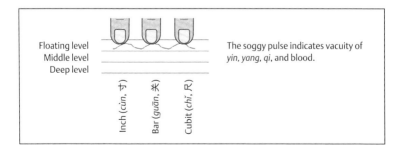

Floating level
Middle level
Deep level

Inch (*cùn*, 寸)
Bar (*guān*, 关)
Cubit (*chǐ*, 尺)

The soggy pulse indicates vacuity of *yin, yang, qi*, and blood.

▨ Pulse Manifestation

- The pulse is located at the superficial level. Its shape is thin and small, with a soft quality.

- The shape of the soggy pulse is thin and small. Its quality is soft. This pulse can only be felt at the superficial level. When the fingers press down with strength, the pulse is imperceptible.

▨ Pulse Principles

- The soggy pulse indicates vacuity of *yin*, *yang*, *qi*, and blood. When the *qi* and blood of the body are depleted, the debilitated *yang qi* lacks the force to move the blood, leading to insufficiency of the strength necessary for blood to charge through the vessels. As a result, the pulse manifests as floating, soft, and forceless.
- When damp evil obstructs the interior, the supply and distribution of *qi* and blood are interrupted. In this case, the pulse can also manifest as soggy.

▨ Differentiation

Soggy pulses are similar to faint and weak pulses in that they are all thin, soft, and forceless pulse manifestations.

▨ Comparing the Pulses

- The soggy pulse is situated at the superficial level. Only light pressure is required to feel it.
- The weak pulse is located at the deep level. It can only be felt with heavy pressure.
- The faint pulse can be felt at the superficial or deep levels. Although thin and soft, it is also indistinct and obscure. It is faintly discernible and vague.

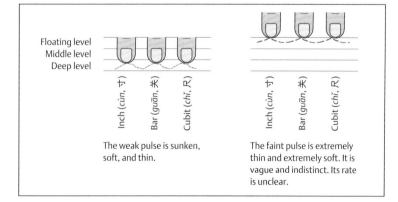

Floating level
Middle level
Deep level

Inch (cùn, 寸)　Bar (guān, 关)　Cubit (chǐ, 尺)

The weak pulse is sunken, soft, and thin.

Inch (cùn, 寸)　Bar (guān, 关)　Cubit (chǐ, 尺)

The faint pulse is extremely thin and extremely soft. It is vague and indistinct. Its rate is unclear.

■ Indications

- The soggy pulse indicates vacuity of *yin*, *yang*, *qi*, and blood.
- The soggy pulse can also indicate damp evil brewing internally. Whenever there is damp evil congesting the interior, it will lead to impairment of the *yang qi* and hindrance of its normal distribution. There will be symptoms such as head heaviness (as if the head is wrapped), phlegm–damp encumbrance, puffy swelling of the skin and flesh, chest oppression, and abdominal distention. A soggy pulse is present in all of these cases.

■ Concurrent Pulses and their Indications

Concurrent Pulse Manifestations	Manifesting Symptoms
Soggy and slow	Vacuity cold
Soggy and rapid	Yin and essence depletion or damp–heat
Soggy and rough	Blood collapse
Soggy and moderate	Cold–damp

The Scattered Pulse (*Sàn Mài*, 散脈)

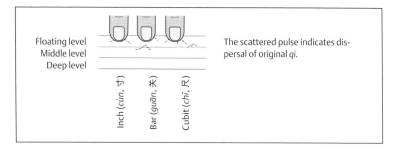

Floating level
Middle level
Deep level

Inch (*cùn*, 寸)
Bar (*guān*, 关)
Cubit (*chǐ*, 尺)

The scattered pulse indicates dispersal of original *qi*.

■ Pulse Manifestation

- The scattered pulse is floating, large, and without root. Its rhythm is uneven.
- The scattered pulse is floating, scattered, and rootless. When palpated at the superficial level, the pulse is sometimes fast and sometimes slow. Its onset and recession are unclear. When palpated with heavy pressure, the pulse is imperceptible.

▦ Pulse Principles

- When the original *qi* of the viscera and bowels is used up, the heart is exhausted and *yang qi* is dispersed, leading to difficulty of the blood circulating properly. As a result, the pulse is floating, scattered, and rootless. It is sometimes fast and sometimes slow, with an uneven rhythm.

▦ Differentiation

The scattered pulse is similar to the soggy, vacuous, and scallion-stalk pulses. They are all floating.

▦ Comparing the Pulses

- The scattered pulse is floating, scattered, and rootless. It has an uneven rhythm.
- The soggy pulse is floating, thin, small, and soft. It has an even rhythm.
- The vacuous pulse is floating and large. Although it is soft and weak at all three levels (superficial, middle, and deep), it has root.
- The scallion-stalk pulse is floating, large, and soft. When the fingers press down lightly to the middle level, the pulse feels hollow.

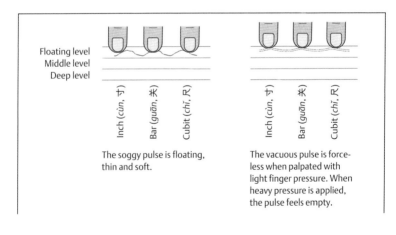

Floating level
Middle level
Deep level

Inch (*cùn*, 寸)　Bar (*guān*, 关)　Cubit (*chǐ*, 尺)

Inch (*cùn*, 寸)　Bar (*guān*, 关)　Cubit (*chǐ*, 尺)

The soggy pulse is floating, thin and soft.

The vacuous pulse is forceless when palpated with light finger pressure. When heavy pressure is applied, the pulse feels empty.

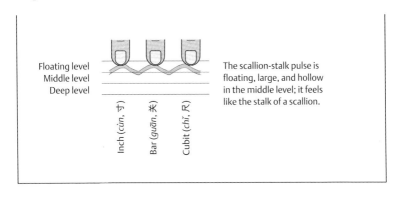

Floating level
Middle level
Deep level

Inch (*cùn*, 寸) Bar (*guān*, 关) Cubit (*chǐ*, 尺)

The scallion-stalk pulse is floating, large, and hollow in the middle level; it feels like the stalk of a scallion.

■ Indications

- The scattered pulse indicates dispersal of the original *qi*. If the body's essence–blood is severely damaged, *yin* and *yang* will separate and be exhausted. As a result, the *qi* and blood of the viscera and bowels will also be consumed, giving rise to a scattered pulse.

The Scallion-stalk Pulse (*Kōu Mài*, 芤脉)

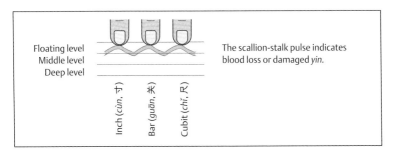

Floating level
Middle level
Deep level

Inch (*cùn*, 寸) Bar (*guān*, 关) Cubit (*chǐ*, 尺)

The scallion-stalk pulse indicates blood loss or damaged *yin*.

■ Pulse Manifestation

- The scallion-stalk pulse is floating, large, and hollow in the middle level; it feels like the stalk of a scallion.
- Under light palpation, the arteries are soft, and the middle level feels hollow. The pulse is large in shape, and it feels exactly like pressing on the stalk of a scallion.

- Since the periphery of the arteries is strong, the center of the arteries then seems forceless in comparison. The pulse is weaker under heavy palpation.

Pulse Principles

- Due to excessive blood loss or great injury to the body fluids, there is a sudden decrease in the blood volume of the body. As a result, there is insufficient *yin*–blood to fill up the arteries, causing it to feel hollow. At this time, since *yang qi* has no *yin* to attach itself to, it will float outwards, forming the scallion-stalk pulse, which is floating, large, and hollow.

Differentiation

The scallion-stalk pulse is similar to the firm and vacuous pulses. All three pulse manifestations are hollow.

Comparing the Pulses

- The scallion-stalk pulse is floating, large, and hollow; it feels like the stalk of a scallion. The surrounding arteries are relatively softer.
- The drumskin pulse is also floating, large, and hollow. However, it is forceful, and feels like the surface of a drum. The surrounding arteries are relatively firmer.
- The vacuous pulse is floating and large. It is forceless at all three levels, yet it still has root.

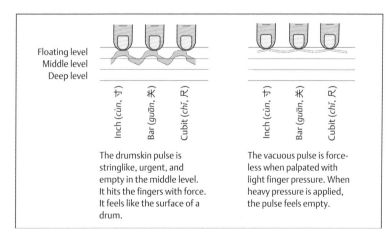

Floating level
Middle level
Deep level

Inch (*cùn*, 寸)   Bar (*guān*, 关)   Cubit (*chǐ*, 尺)

Inch (*cùn*, 寸)   Bar (*guān*, 关)   Cubit (*chǐ*, 尺)

The drumskin pulse is stringlike, urgent, and empty in the middle level. It hits the fingers with force. It feels like the surface of a drum.

The vacuous pulse is forceless when palpated with light finger pressure. When heavy pressure is applied, the pulse feels empty.

▨ Indications

- The scallion-stalk pulse indicates blood loss or consumption of *yin* humor, such as in cases of blood ejection, flooding (*bēng zhōng*, 崩中), bloody urine, or other bleeding disorders; or if there is vomiting, diarrhea, and great sweating (*dà hàn*, 大汗). All of the above cause great damage to the body fluids, giving rise to a scallion-stalk pulse.

▨ Concurrent Pulses and their Indications

Concurrent Pulse Manifestations	Manifesting Symptoms
Floating and scallion-stalk	Damage to both *qi* and *yin*
Scallion-stalk and rapid	*Yin* vacuity
Scallion-stalk and vacuous	Blood collapse and seminal loss
Scallion-stalk and slow	Blood loss and right *qi* vacuity

The Drumskin Pulse (*Gé Mài*, 革脉)

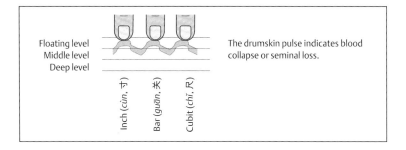

Floating level
Middle level
Deep level

Inch (*cùn*, 寸)
Bar (*guān*, 关)
Cubit (*chǐ*, 尺)

The drumskin pulse indicates blood collapse or seminal loss.

▨ Pulse Manifestation

- It is floating and hollow, and feels like the surface of a drum.
- The drumskin pulse is stringlike, urgent, and empty in the middle level. It feels like the surface of a drum.

▨ Pulse Principles

- When the essence–blood of the body is severely depleted, there will be insufficient *yin* blood to fill up the arteries, and thus the arteries feel hollow. At this time, since *yang* qi has no *yin* to attach itself to, it will float outwards, forming the drumskin pulse, which is floating, large, and hollow.
- Generally speaking, the firm pulse is stronger and more forceful than the scallion-stalk pulse, indicating that the *yang* qi in the case of the drumskin pulse is much stronger than that of the scallion-stalk pulse.

▨ Differentiation

The firm pulse is similar to the scallion-stalk and vacuous pulses. All three pulse manifestations are hollow.

▨ Comparing the Pulses

- The drumskin pulse is floating, large, and hollow. It hits the fingers with force, and feels like the surface of a drum. The surrounding arteries are relatively firmer.
- The scallion-stalk pulse is floating, large, and hollow. It feels like the stalk of a scallion. The surrounding arteries are relatively softer.

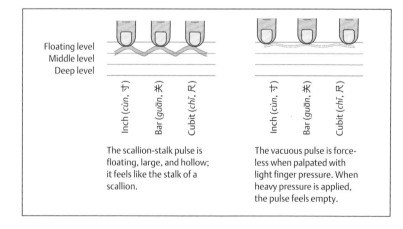

The scallion-stalk pulse is floating, large, and hollow; it feels like the stalk of a scallion.

The vacuous pulse is forceless when palpated with light finger pressure. When heavy pressure is applied, the pulse feels empty.

Indications

- The drumskin pulse indicates signs and symptoms of blood collapse or seminal loss. When *qi* and blood are depleted and semen has been severely wasted, this will manifest as a drumskin pulse.

The Sunken Pulse (*Chén Mài,* 沉脉)

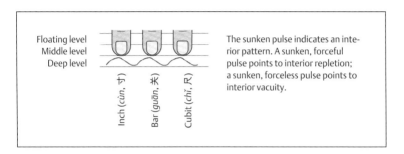

Floating level
Middle level
Deep level

Inch (*cùn,* 寸)
Bar (*guān,* 关)
Cubit (*chǐ,* 尺)

The sunken pulse indicates an interior pattern. A sunken, forceful pulse points to interior repletion; a sunken, forceless pulse points to interior vacuity.

Pulse Manifestation

- It can only be felt when palpated with heavy finger pressure.
- The sunken pulse is not very prominent at the superficial and middle levels. The pulse can only be felt when the fingers press down to the level of the sinews and bones.

Pulse Principles

- **Interior repletion pattern:** When disease evil enters the interior, the body is able to resist the disease via the battle between right *qi* and evil *qi* if the patient's *qi* and blood are abundant. This will cause the pulse to be sunken and forceful. This pattern is called an interior repletion pattern.
- **Interior vacuity pattern:** If the patient's *qi* and blood are depleted, the distribution of *qi* and blood is impaired, giving rise to a sunken and forceless pulse. This is called an interior vacuity pattern.

Differentiation

The sunken pulse is similar to the hidden, firm, and weak pulses. They are all located at the deep level, and can only be felt with heavy palpation.

Comparing the Pulses

- The sunken pulse is located at the level of the bones and sinews, and can only be felt with heavy palpation.
- The hidden pulse is deeper than the sunken pulse, located within the bones and sinews, and therefore cannot be felt with moderate palpation. The fingers must stick close to the bones and sinews to be able to feel the pulse.
- The firm pulse is similar to the sunken pulse, but its shape is longer and more stringlike. It is also attached to the surface of the bones and sinews. It is firm and steadfast.
- The weak pulse is also found at the deep level. It is soft and forceless.

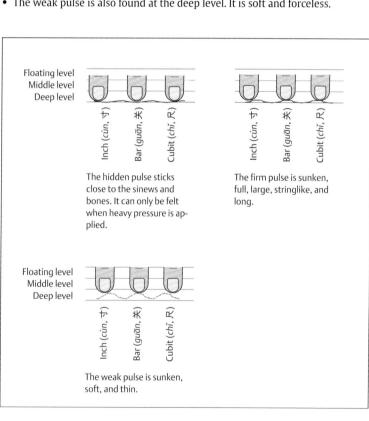

The hidden pulse sticks close to the sinews and bones. It can only be felt when heavy pressure is applied.

The firm pulse is sunken, full, large, stringlike, and long.

The weak pulse is sunken, soft, and thin.

▦ Indications

- The sunken pulse indicates an interior pattern. A sunken, forceful pulse points to an interior repletion pattern, and is commonly seen in phlegm–food, *qi* stagnation, accumulation and stagnation of cold evil, dysentery, or edema.
- A sunken, forceless pulse points to interior vacuity pattern, commonly seen in *qi* and blood vacuity or *yang qi* debilitation.

▦ Concurrent Pulses and their Indications

Concurrent Pulse Manifestations	Manifesting Symptoms
Sunken and slow	Interior cold
Sunken and rapid	Interior heat
Sunken and moderate	Water–damp
Sunken and rough	*Qi* depression
Sunken and slippery	Phlegm–food or damp–heat
Sunken and stringlike	Internal pain
Sunken and tight	Cold pain

The Hidden Pulse (*Fú Mài*, 伏脉)

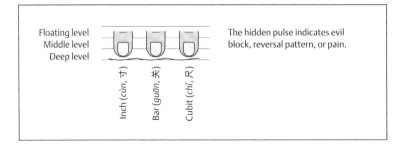

Floating level
Middle level
Deep level

Inch (*cùn*, 寸)
Bar (*guān*, 关)
Cubit (*chǐ*, 尺)

The hidden pulse indicates evil block, reversal pattern, or pain.

Pulse Manifestation

- The hidden pulse sticks close to the sinews and bones. It can only be felt when heavy pressure is applied.
- The hidden pulse is located within the sinews and bones, and cannot be felt with just moderately heavy palpation. The fingers must stick close to the sinews and bones in order to feel the pulse manifestation.

Pulse Principles

- When evil *qi* in the body becomes intense, it can easily obstruct the circulation of *qi* and blood, leading to inability of the pulse *qi* to move in its normal manner. This results in a hidden pulse.
- If chronic intractable illness debilitates the right *qi*, there will be insufficient *yang qi* to arouse the blood vessels. This can also give rise to a hidden pulse.

Differentiation

The hidden pulse is similar to the sunken pulse.

Comparing the Pulses

- The depth of the hidden pulse is deeper than that of the sunken pulse. It is almost adherent to the sinews and bones.
- The sunken pulse is not very prominent at the superficial and middle levels. Only when the fingers press down to the level of the sinews and bones can the pulse be felt.

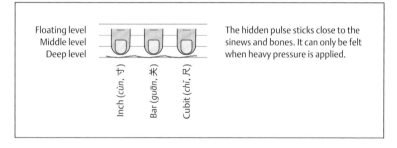

Floating level
Middle level
Deep level

Inch (*cùn*, 寸)   Bar (*guān*, 关)   Cubit (*chǐ*, 尺)

The hidden pulse sticks close to the sinews and bones. It can only be felt when heavy pressure is applied.

▦ Indications

- The hidden pulse indicates evil block (*xié bì*, 邪閉), reversal pattern (*jué zhèng*, 厥證), or pain. A hidden pulse is likely to manifest whenever there is repletion evil hidden internally, such as *qi* block, cold block, heat block, fire block, severe pain, accumulations and gatherings from the accumulation of lumps in the abdomen leading to visceral pain, lodged rheum (*liú yǐn*, 留飲) from long-term fluid retention, poor digestion, abiding food (*sù shí*, 宿食) from food retention in the stomach, or sudden turmoil (*huò luàn*, 霍亂) with vomiting and dysentery.
- The hidden pulse can also indicate debilitation of *yang*. If there is debilitation of heart *yang* or *yang qi* on the verge of expiration with a clouded spirit and reverse-flow (*jué nì*, 厥逆), a hidden and forceless pulse will manifest.

The Firm Pulse (*Láo Mài*, 牢脈)

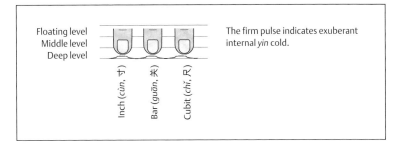

Floating level
Middle level
Deep level

Inch (*cùn*, 寸)
Bar (*guān*, 关)
Cubit (*chǐ*, 尺)

The firm pulse indicates exuberant internal *yin* cold.

▦ Pulse Manifestation

- With heavy palpation, the pulse feels full, large, stringlike, and long.
- The firm pulse adheres to the sinews and bones, and is firm and steadfast; therefore, the shape of the pulse is comparatively longer and more stringlike than normal.

▦ Pulse Principles

- Since cold evil by nature causes contraction, tautness, congealing, and stagnation, *yang qi* will become hidden and have difficulty rising and expanding when there is exuberant *yin* cold in the body. This will result in a firm pulse that is sunken, stringlike, long, and steadfast.

▥ **Differentiation**

The firm pulse is similar to the sunken and hidden pulses.

▥ **Comparing the Pulses**

- The depth of the firm pulse is deeper than that of the sunken pulse. It is almost adherent to the sinews and bones, and has a fixed and determined rhythm. Relatively speaking, however, the depth of the firm pulse is still not as deep as that of the hidden pulse.

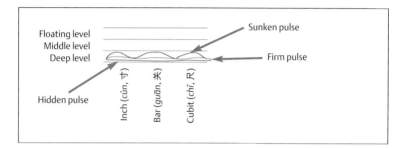

▥ **Indications**

- The firm pulse indicates exuberance of *yin* cold in the body, which includes signs and symptoms such as pain in the heart region and abdomen, and wind tetany with hypertonicity. These signs and symptoms are usually accompanied by a firm pulse.

The Weak Pulse (*Ruò Mài,* 弱脉)

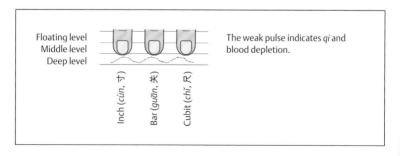

▨ Pulse Manifestation

- The pulse is sunken, thin, and extremely soft.
- The weak pulse cannot be felt with light palpation; heavy finger pressure is required to feel the pulse. It is soft and forceless.

▨ Pulse Principles

- When there is insufficient *qi* and blood in the body, the blood is unable to fill the vessels, and *yang qi* lacks the force to propel blood to circulate, resulting in the manifestation of a weak pulse that is sunken, thin, and soft.

▨ Differentiation

The weak pulse is similar to the soggy and faint pulses. All of these pulse types are thin, soft, and forceless.

▨ Comparing the Pulses

- The weak pulse is found at the deep level.
- The soggy pulse is found at the superficial level.
- The faint pulse can be found at either the superficial or deep level. The pulse manifestation is vague and indistinct, as if it is sometimes present and sometimes absent, and occasionally it feels as if it is on the verge of expiry.
- The shape of the fine pulse is thin, small, and very clear and distinct. Unlike the faint pulse, it is neither vague nor indistinct.

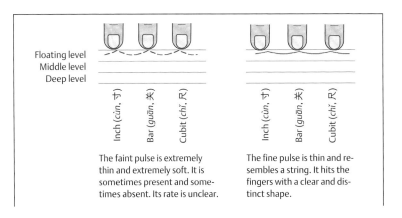

Floating level
Middle level
Deep level

Inch (*cùn*, 寸)   Bar (*guān*, 关)   Cubit (*chǐ*, 尺)

Inch (*cùn*, 寸)   Bar (*guān*, 关)   Cubit (*chǐ*, 尺)

The faint pulse is extremely thin and extremely soft. It is sometimes present and sometimes absent. Its rate is unclear.

The fine pulse is thin and resembles a string. It hits the fingers with a clear and distinct shape.

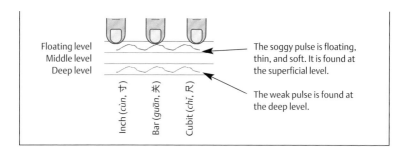

Floating level
Middle level
Deep level

Inch (cùn, 寸)   Bar (guān, 关)   Cubit (chǐ, 尺)

The soggy pulse is floating, thin, and soft. It is found at the superficial level.

The weak pulse is found at the deep level.

▩ Indications

- The weak pulse indicates *qi* and blood depletion. In cases of chronic and intractable illness causing damage to original *qi*, blood collapse due to seminal loss, enduring cough due to vacuity taxation, spleen deficiency, diarrhea, poor intake of food due to stomach weakness, or weakness and wilting of the sinews and bones, the pulse will be weak.

▩ Concurrent Pulses and their Indications

Concurrent Pulse Manifestations	Manifesting Symptoms
Rough and weak	Blood vacuity or blood stasis
Weak and faint	Debilitation of *qi*
Weak and rapid	*Yin* vacuity or blood vacuity

The Slow Pulse (*Chí Mài*, 遲脈)

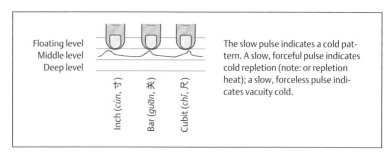

Floating level
Middle level
Deep level

Inch (cùn, 寸)   Bar (guān, 关)   Cubit (chǐ, 尺)

The slow pulse indicates a cold pattern. A slow, forceful pulse indicates cold repletion (note: or repletion heat); a slow, forceless pulse indicates vacuity cold.

▦ Pulse Manifestation

- The onset of the pulse is slow and moderate. There are three beats per respiration.
- The pulse of a person of normal health beats four to five times per respiration, whereas the slow pulse beats only three times per respiration. In addition, the slow pulse can be felt with light or heavy pressure.

▦ Pulse Principles

- The slow pulse not only indicates a cold pattern, but can also indicate a heat pattern. This is because when cold or heat evil in the body is intensified, *qi* and blood circulation will be impeded. Furthermore, if the pulse is slow and forceless, this indicates a vacuity cold pattern; if the pulse is slow and forceful, this denotes a cold repletion pattern. Therefore, one must determine the significance of a slow pulse with caution.

▦ Differentiation

The slow pulse is similar to the moderate and rough pulses. All three pulse types are slightly slower than normal.

▦ Comparing the Pulses

- The slow pulse beats three times per respiration.
- The moderate pulse is slightly faster than the slow pulse. It beats four times per respiration.
- The shape of the rough pulse is short and abnormally thin. Its onset is harsh, causing its rate to be slightly slower than normal.

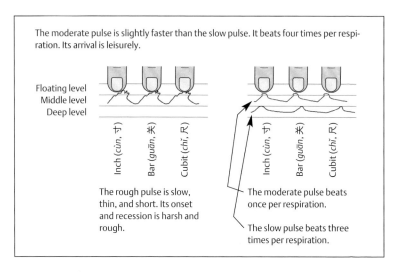

The moderate pulse is slightly faster than the slow pulse. It beats four times per respiration. Its arrival is leisurely.

Floating level
Middle level
Deep level

Inch (cùn, 寸)
Bar (guān, 关)
Cubit (chǐ, 尺)

Inch (cùn, 寸)
Bar (guān, 关)
Cubit (chǐ, 尺)

The rough pulse is slow, thin, and short. Its onset and recession is harsh and rough.

The moderate pulse beats once per respiration.

The slow pulse beats three times per respiration.

■ Indications

- The slow pulse indicates a cold pattern. A slow, forceful pulse indicates cold repletion (note: or repletion heat); a slow, forceless pulse indicates vacuity cold.
- The slow pulse can also indicate a heat pattern. This is because when there is congestion of heat evil in the body, blood flow within the arteries is inhibited, which leads to stasis and heat contending with each other and binding to the blood chamber, giving rise to a slow pulse.

■ Concurrent Pulses and their Indications

Concurrent Pulse Manifestations	Manifesting Symptoms
Floating and slow	Exterior cold
Sunken and slow	Interior cold
Slow and slippery	Phlegm–rheum
Slow and rough	Blood stasis or blood vacuity
Slow and fine	*Qi* vacuity

The Moderate Pulse (*Huǎn Mài*, 緩脈)

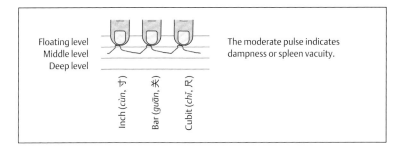

Floating level
Middle level
Deep level

Inch (*cùn*, 寸)
Bar (*guān*, 关)
Cubit (*chǐ*, 尺)

The moderate pulse indicates dampness or spleen vacuity.

▦ Pulse Manifestation

- The moderate pulse beats four times per respiration. Its arrival is leisurely.
- The moderate pulse is slightly faster than the slow pulse. It beats four times per respiration. The moderate pulse can be felt with either light or heavy pressure.

▦ Pulse Principles

- When there is spleen *qi* vacuity or internal encumbrance of damp evil, the circulation of *qi* and blood will be obstructed, and there will be insufficient *qi* and blood to fill up the arteries. This results in a moderate pulse.

▦ Differentiation

The moderate pulse is similar to the slow and rough pulses.

▦ Comparing the Pulses

- The weak pulse is found at the deep level.
- The soggy pulse is found at the superficial level.
- The shape of the rough pulse is short and abnormally thin, with a harsh onset and recession. For these reasons, the pulse rate is slower than normal.

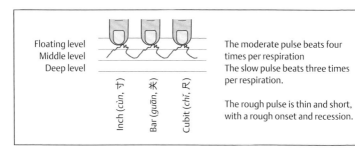

Floating level
Middle level
Deep level

Inch (cùn, 寸) Bar (guān, 关) Cubit (chǐ, 尺)

The moderate pulse beats four times per respiration
The slow pulse beats three times per respiration.

The rough pulse is thin and short, with a rough onset and recession.

▨ Indications

• The moderate pulse indicates damp evil accumulating and stagnating in the interior, or detriment of spleen *qi* vacuity.

▨ Concurrent Pulses and their Indications

Concurrent Pulse Manifestations	Manifesting Symptoms
Floating and moderate	Wind damage or wind–damp
Sunken and moderate	Cold–damp or damp impediment
Moderate and slippery	Spleen heat
Moderate and weak	*Qi* vacuity

The Rough Pulse (*Sè Mài*, 涩脉)

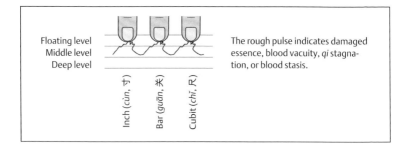

Floating level
Middle level
Deep level

Inch (cùn, 寸) Bar (guān, 关) Cubit (chǐ, 尺)

The rough pulse indicates damaged essence, blood vacuity, *qi* stagnation, or blood stasis.

Pulse Manifestation

- The rough pulse is slow, thin, and short. Its onset and recession are harsh. It is extremely coarse.
- The shape of the rough pulse is thin and short. It feels like a light knife scraping on bamboo. It has a harsh onset and recession, and is extremely coarse.

Pulse Principles

- When *qi* and blood circulation is obstructed due to damaged essence, blood vacuity, *qi* stagnation, or blood stasis, the arrival and departure of the pulse *qi* will be harsh and coarse. This results in a rough pulse.

Differentiation

The rough pulse is similar to the bound pulse. Both pulse manifestations are relatively sluggish.

Comparing the Pulses

- The rough pulse feels sluggish because it is unsmooth with a harsh and coarse onset and recession.
- The bound pulse is also sluggish. Although it does not have a rough onset and recession, it pauses suddenly at irregular intervals.

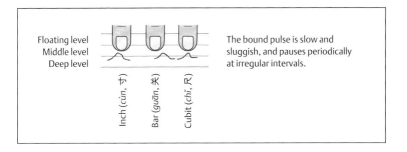

Floating level
Middle level
Deep level

Inch (*cùn*, 寸)
Bar (*guān*, 关)
Cubit (*chǐ*, 尺)

The bound pulse is slow and sluggish, and pauses periodically at irregular intervals.

Indications

- The rough pulse indicates damaged essence, blood vacuity, *qi* stagnation, or blood stasis.

The Bound Pulse (*Jié Mài*, 結脈)

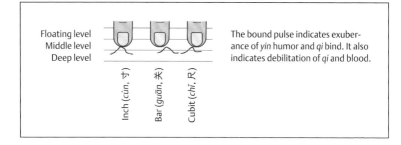

Floating level
Middle level
Deep level

Inch (*cùn*, 寸)
Bar (*guān*, 关)
Cubit (*chǐ*, 尺)

The bound pulse indicates exuberance of *yin* humor and *qi* bind. It also indicates debilitation of *qi* and blood.

▦ Pulse Manifestation

- The bound pulse is slow and sluggish, and pauses periodically at irregular intervals.
- The rate of the bound pulse is sluggish. Occasionally, it skips a beat and then starts up again. The skips occur at irregular intervals.

▦ Pulse Principles

- If there is static blood, phlegm–rheum, abiding food, or *qi* stagnation obstructing the flow of *qi* and blood, this will lead to an exuberance of *yin* humor and cause *yang qi* to become hidden, resulting in a bound pulse that is sluggish and skips at irregular intervals.

▦ Differentiation

The bound pulse is similar to the skipping and intermittent pulses. These three pulse types all show sudden interruptions.

▦ Comparing the Pulses

- The bound pulse is sluggish and skips a beat at irregular intervals. The duration of each pause is relatively short.
- The skipping pulse is urgent and rapid. It also skips a beat at irregular intervals. The duration of each pause is relatively short.
- The intermittent pulse is more sluggish than the skipping pulse. It pauses at regular intervals, each pause being of relatively long duration.

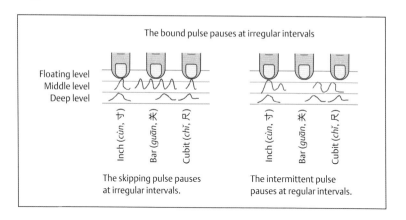

The bound pulse pauses at irregular intervals

Floating level
Middle level
Deep level

Inch (cùn, 寸)   Bar (guān, 关)   Cubit (chǐ, 尺)

The skipping pulse pauses at irregular intervals.

The intermittent pulse pauses at regular intervals.

■ Indications

- **A bound pulse that is forceful:** The bound pulse indicates the exuberance of *yin* humor and congestion of the *qi* dynamic. Signs and symptoms include those of blood stasis, phlegm–rheum, abiding food, and *qi* depression.
- **A bound pulse that is forceless:** The bound pulse can also indicate *qi* and blood debilitation. Signs and symptoms include vacuity taxation leading to illness and chronic intractable disease.

The Rapid Pulse (*Shuò Mài*, 數脈)

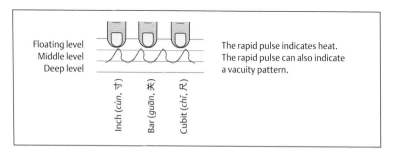

Floating level
Middle level
Deep level

Inch (cùn, 寸)   Bar (guān, 关)   Cubit (chǐ, 尺)

The rapid pulse indicates heat. The rapid pulse can also indicate a vacuity pattern.

Pulse Manifestation

- The rapid pulse beats five or more times per respiration.
- The rapid pulse beats more quickly than normal. During one respiration (one inhalation and one exhalation), the pulse beats five or more times. Its rate is 90 or more beats per minute.

Pulse Principles

- When evil heat intensifies in the body, it will scorch and damage the *yin* humor and cause hyperactivity of *yang qi*. The movement of *qi* and blood will speed up tremendously, giving rise to a rapid pulse.
- If a patient has severe *yin* vacuity, the *yin* depletion will lead to the internal generation of vacuity heat. In this case, the pulse will be rapid, vacuous, and forceless.

Differentiation

The rapid pulse is similar to the racing, slippery, and stirred pulses. All four pulses are relatively fast.

Comparing the Pulses

- The rapid pulse beats five or more times per respiration.
- The racing pulse is faster than the rapid pulse. It beats seven to eight (or more) times per respiration, totaling 140 or more beats per minute.
- The stirred pulse is smooth and evasive, like a bean. It is slippery, rapid, and forceful. It oscillates and feels unstable.
- The slippery pulse has an extremely smooth onset and recession. Its shape is round and smooth, and feels like pearls rolling on a dish.

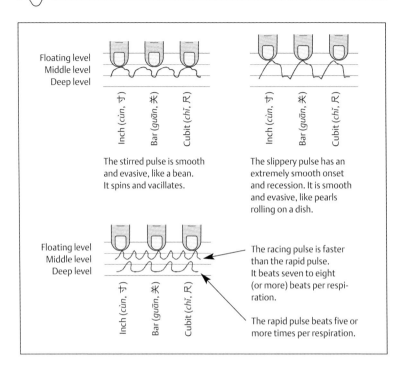

The stirred pulse is smooth and evasive, like a bean. It spins and vacillates.

The slippery pulse has an extremely smooth onset and recession. It is smooth and evasive, like pearls rolling on a dish.

The racing pulse is faster than the rapid pulse. It beats seven to eight (or more) beats per respiration.

The rapid pulse beats five or more times per respiration.

▧ Indications

- The rapid pulse indicates heat brewing in the interior, which is present in patterns such as stomach heat with swift digestion, intestinal heat with diarrhea, welling-abscess (*yōng*, 癰) of the lung and intestines, external contraction of evil heat, or effulgent *yin* vacuity fire. All of these can lead to a rapid pulse.
- The rapid pulse can also indicate a vacuity pattern. Signs and symptoms of vacuity taxation and depletion can give rise to a rapid pulse; however, the pulse will manifest as rapid and forceless.

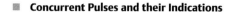

Concurrent Pulses and their Indications

Concurrent Pulse Manifestations	Manifesting Symptoms
Floating and rapid	Exterior heat
Sunken and rapid	Interior heat
Rapid and surging	Exuberant heat
Fine and rapid	*Yin* vacuity internal heat
Rapid and stringlike or rapid and slippery	Liver–fire or phlegm–heat

The Racing Pulse (*Jí Mài*, 疾脈)

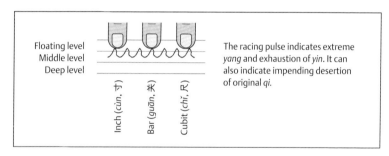

Floating level
Middle level
Deep level

Inch (*cùn*, 寸) Bar (*guān*, 关) Cubit (*chǐ*, 尺)

The racing pulse indicates extreme *yang* and exhaustion of *yin*. It can also indicate impending desertion of original *qi*.

Pulse Manifestation

- The racing pulse beats seven or eight times per respiration; the arrival of the pulse is hurried.
- The rate of the racing pulse is very fast. It beats seven to eight (or more) times per respiration, totaling 140 or more beats per minute.

Pulse Principles

- When repletion heat in the body is intensified, heat evil will scorch and damage the *yin* humor to cause hyperactivity of *yang qi*. This gives rise to a racing pulse.
- When there is a vacuity pattern with desiccation of *yin* humor, *yang qi* will lack the anchor to attach itself to, and will thus float outward. In this case, there will be a racing pulse that is forceless.

■ Differentiation

The racing pulse is similar to the rapid, slippery, and stirred pulses.

■ Comparing the Pulses

- The rate of the racing pulse is faster than that of the rapid pulse. It beats seven to eight (or more) times per respiration, totaling 140 or more beats per minute.
- The rapid pulse beats five or more times per respiration.
- The stirred pulse is smooth and evasive like a bean. The pulse manifestation is slippery, rapid, and forceful. It oscillates and feels unstable.
- The slippery pulse has an extremely smooth onset and recession. Its shape is round and smooth, and feels like pearls rolling on a dish.

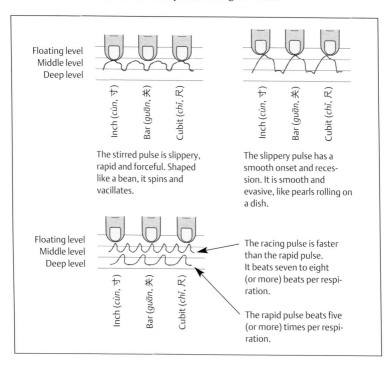

The stirred pulse is slippery, rapid and forceful. Shaped like a bean, it spins and vacillates.

The slippery pulse has a smooth onset and recession. It is smooth and evasive, like pearls rolling on a dish.

The racing pulse is faster than the rapid pulse. It beats seven to eight (or more) beats per respiration.

The rapid pulse beats five (or more) times per respiration.

Indications

The racing pulse indicates extreme *yang* and exhaustion of *yin*. It can also indicate impending desertion of original *qi*.

The Skipping Pulse (*Cù Mài*, 促脉)

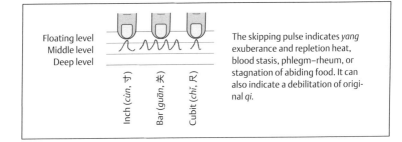

Floating level
Middle level
Deep level

Inch (*cùn*, 寸)   Bar (*guān*, 关)   Cubit (*chǐ*, 尺)

The skipping pulse indicates *yang* exuberance and repletion heat, blood stasis, phlegm–rheum, or stagnation of abiding food. It can also indicate a debilitation of original *qi*.

Pulse Manifestation

- The skipping pulse is rapid and pauses periodically with an indeterminate rhythm (skips at irregular intervals).
- The skipping pulse is urgent and rapid. It skips a beat at irregular intervals, but the duration of each pause is relatively short.

Pulse Principles

- When factors such as static blood, phlegm–rheum, or abiding food obstruct the flow of the *qi* dynamic, or when heat evil is so intense that it causes hyperactivity of *yang qi*, the *yin* and *yang* of the body will be in disharmony, and the pulse will be skipping (hurried with sudden interruptions).

Differentiation

The skipping pulse is similar to the bound and intermittent pulses. All three pulses show sudden interruptions.

Comparing the Pulses

- The skipping pulse is urgent and rapid. It skips a beat at irregular intervals. Each pause is of relatively short duration.

- The bound pulse is sluggish and skips a beat at irregular intervals. The duration of each pause is relatively short.
- The intermittent pulse is more sluggish than the skipping pulse. It pauses at regular intervals, with each pause being of relatively long duration.

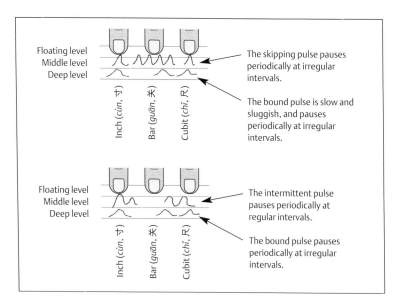

Indications

The skipping pulse indicates exuberance of *yang qi*, heat brewing in the interior, blood stasis, phlegm–rheum, or stagnation of abiding food. The skipping pulse can also indicate debilitation of original *qi*.

Concurrent Pulses and their Indications

Concurrent Pulse Manifestations	Manifesting Symptoms
Floating and skipping	*Yang* brightness warm disease
Skipping and forceful	Repletion evil depressed heat
Skipping and forceless	Debilitation of the true origin

The Stirred Pulse (*Dòng Mài*, 動脈)

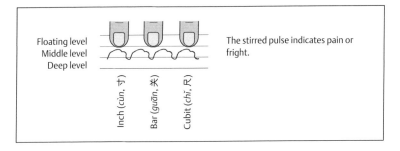

Floating level
Middle level
Deep level

Inch (*cùn*, 寸)
Bar (*guān*, 关)
Cubit (*chǐ*, 尺)

The stirred pulse indicates pain or fright.

Pulse Manifestation

- The stirred pulse is slippery, rapid and forceful. Shaped like a bean, it spins and vacillates.
- The shape of the stirred pulse is smooth and evasive, like a bean. It is slippery, rapid, and forceful. It oscillates and feels unstable.

Pulse Principles

- When there is pain due to static blood or *qi* stagnation, *yin* and *yang* will easily fall out of harmony. When there is fright, fear, and flusteredness, *qi* and blood will be chaotic. All of these factors impair the normal ascent and descent of *qi* and blood, thus producing a stirred pulse.

Differentiation

The stirred pulse is similar to the rapid, racing, and slippery pulses. These four pulses are all relatively fast.

Comparing the Pulses

- The stirred pulse is smooth and evasive like a bean. It is slippery, rapid, and forceful. It oscillates and feels unstable.
- The rapid pulse beats five or more times per respiration.
- The racing pulse is faster than the rapid pulse. It beats seven to eight (or more) times per respiration, totaling 140 or more beats per minute.
- The slippery pulse has an extremely smooth onset and recession. Its shape is round and smooth, and feels like pearls rolling on a dish.

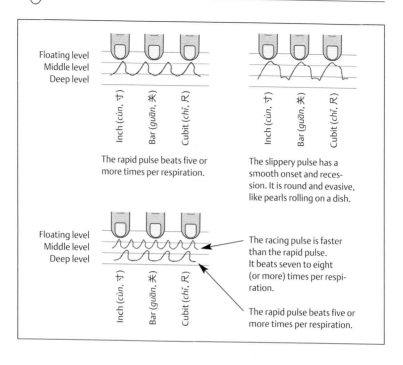

Floating level
Middle level
Deep level

Inch (*cùn*, 寸)   Bar (*guān*, 关)   Cubit (*chǐ*, 尺)

The rapid pulse beats five or more times per respiration.

Inch (*cùn*, 寸)   Bar (*guān*, 关)   Cubit (*chǐ*, 尺)

The slippery pulse has a smooth onset and recession. It is round and evasive, like pearls rolling on a dish.

Floating level
Middle level
Deep level

Inch (*cùn*, 寸)   Bar (*guān*, 关)   Cubit (*chǐ*, 尺)

The racing pulse is faster than the rapid pulse. It beats seven to eight (or more) times per respiration.

The rapid pulse beats five or more times per respiration.

■ **Indications**

• The stirred pulse indicates pain due to blood stasis or *qi* stagnation. It can also indicate fright palpitations in the heart.

■ **Concurrent Pulses and their Indications**

Concurrent Pulse Manifestations	Manifesting Symptoms
Stirred and weak	Fright palpitations
Stirred and rapid	Heat
Stirred and replete	Pain
Stirred and slippery	Phlegm–damp

The Vacuous Pulse (*Xū Mài*, 虚脉)

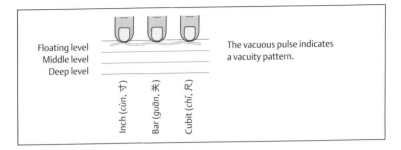

Floating level
Middle level
Deep level

Inch (cùn, 寸)
Bar (guān, 夫)
Cubit (chǐ, 尺)

The vacuous pulse indicates a vacuity pattern.

▦ Pulse Manifestation

- The vacuous pulse is forceless when palpated with light finger pressure. Under heavy finger pressure, the pulse feels empty.
- Regardless of the level of palpation, the vacuous pulse is soft, weak, and forceless. Its shape is thin and small, and feels hollow.

▦ Pulse Principles

- When *yang qi* is debilitated, the force that propels blood circulation is weakened, thus producing a vacuous pulse that is soft, weak, and forceless.
- When there is insufficient blood, *yang qi* will not have an anchor to attach itself to and will therefore float outward. This will produce a vacuous pulse that is large and soft.

▦ Differentiation

The vacuous pulse is similar to the scallion-stalk, soggy, and scattered pulses. The main characteristic of these pulse manifestations is that they are all located in the shallow part of the fleshy exterior.

▦ Comparing the Pulses

- Regardless of the level of palpation, the vacuous pulse is soft, weak, and forceless. Its shape is thin and small, and feels hollow.
- The shape of the floating pulse is neither large nor small. The strength of the floating pulse is most prominent under light palpation. Although its

strength is slightly reduced when heavy pressure is applied, it does not feel empty.

- The scallion-stalk pulse is found at the superficial level. Its shape is very large and hollow. It has the same hollow sensation as the stalk of a scallion.
- The soggy pulse is found at the superficial level. Its shape is thin, small, and soft.
- The scattered pulse is found at the superficial level. It is chaotic as if it has no root. Its shape is thin and small. It has an uneven rhythm.

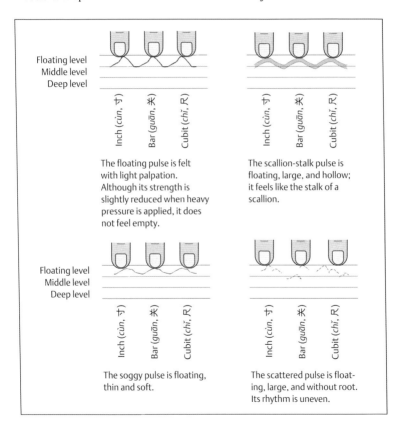

Floating level
Middle level
Deep level

Inch (*cùn*, 寸)   Bar (*guān*, 关)   Cubit (*chǐ*, 尺)

The floating pulse is felt with light palpation. Although its strength is slightly reduced when heavy pressure is applied, it does not feel empty.

Inch (*cùn*, 寸)   Bar (*guān*, 关)   Cubit (*chǐ*, 尺)

The scallion-stalk pulse is floating, large, and hollow; it feels like the stalk of a scallion.

Floating level
Middle level
Deep level

Inch (*cùn*, 寸)   Bar (*guān*, 关)   Cubit (*chǐ*, 尺)

The soggy pulse is floating, thin and soft.

Inch (*cùn*, 寸)   Bar (*guān*, 关)   Cubit (*chǐ*, 尺)

The scattered pulse is floating, large, and without root. Its rhythm is uneven.

Indications

The vacuous pulse indicates *qi* and blood vacuity or depletion of original *qi*.

■ **Concurrent Pulses and their Indications**

Concurrent Pulse Manifestations	Manifesting Symptoms
Floating and vacuous	*Qi* vacuity
Sunken and vacuous	Interior vacuity
Vacuous and rough	Blood vacuity
Vacuous and rapid	*Yin* vacuity
Vacuous and slow	Vacuity cold

The Faint Pulse (*Wēi Mài*, 微脉)

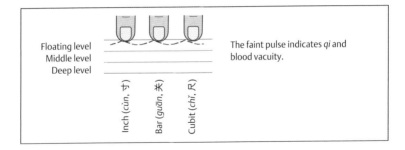

Floating level
Middle level
Deep level

Inch (*cùn*, 寸)   Bar (*guān*, 关)   Cubit (*chǐ*, 尺)

The faint pulse indicates *qi* and blood vacuity.

■ **Pulse Manifestation**

- The faint pulse is extremely thin and extremely soft. It is vague and indistinct, and has an unclear rate.
- The faint pulse can be found at the superficial or deep level. The pulse manifestation is vague and indistinct, as if it is sometimes present and sometimes absent, and it occasionally feels as if it is on the verge of expiry.

■ **Pulse Principles**

- When *yang qi* or *yin qi* is severely depleted, there will be insufficient *yang qi* to propel the circulation of blood, and there will not be enough blood to fill up the arteries. This will result in a faint pulse that is vague and indistinct, as if it is sometimes present and sometimes absent, and it occasionally feels as if it is on the verge of expiry.

Differentiation

The faint pulse is similar to the soggy and fine pulses. These pulses are all thin, soft, and forceless.

Comparing the Pulses

- The faint pulse can be felt at either the superficial or the deep level. The pulse manifestation is vague and indistinct, as if it is sometimes present and sometimes absent, and it occasionally feels as if it is on the verge of expiry.
- The weak pulse is found at the deep level.
- The soggy pulse is found at the superficial level.
- The shape of the fine pulse is thin, small, and very clear and distinct. Unlike the faint pulse, it is neither vague nor indistinct.

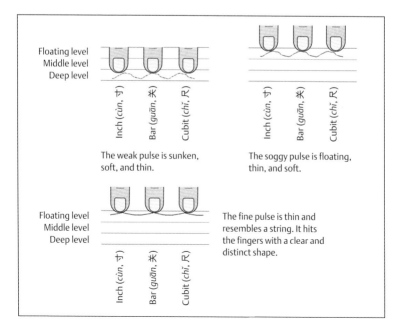

The weak pulse is sunken, soft, and thin.

The soggy pulse is floating, thin, and soft.

The fine pulse is thin and resembles a string. It hits the fingers with a clear and distinct shape.

Indications

- The faint pulse indicates depletion of visceral and bowel *qi*.

Concurrent Pulses and their Indications

Concurrent Pulse Manifestations	Manifesting Symptoms
Floating and faint	Debilitation of *qi*
Sunken and faint	*Yin* vacuity
Faint and rough	Blood collapse

The Fine Pulse (*Xì Mài*, 細脈)

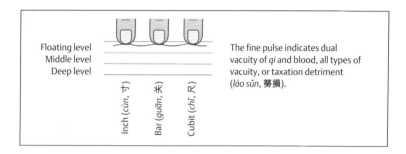

Floating level
Middle level
Deep level

Inch (*cùn*, 寸)   Bar (*guān*, 关)   Cubit (*chǐ*, 尺)

The fine pulse indicates dual vacuity of *qi* and blood, all types of vacuity, or taxation detriment (*láo sǔn*, 笭損).

Pulse Manifestation

- The fine pulse is thin (like a thread) yet clear.
- The shape of the fine pulse is thin, small, and very clear and distinct. Unlike the faint pulse, it is neither vague nor indistinct.

Pulse Principles

- When *qi* and blood are depleted, there is insufficient blood to fill up the arteries and insufficient *yang qi* to circulate the blood. This results in a fine pulse.
- When there is internal obstruction of damp evil or heat evil deeply entering the construction and defense (*yíng wèi*, 營衛), the pulse will be fine.

■ **Differentiation**

The fine pulse is similar to the weak, soggy, and faint pulses. They are all thin, soft, and forceless.

■ **Comparing the Pulses**

- The shape of the fine pulse is thin, small, and very clear and distinct. Unlike the faint pulse, it is neither vague nor indistinct.
- The weak pulse is found at the deep level.
- The soggy pulse is found at the superficial level.
- The faint pulse can be felt at either the superficial or deep level. The pulse manifestation is vague and indistinct, as if it is sometimes present and sometimes absent, and it occasionally feels as if it is on the verge of expiry.

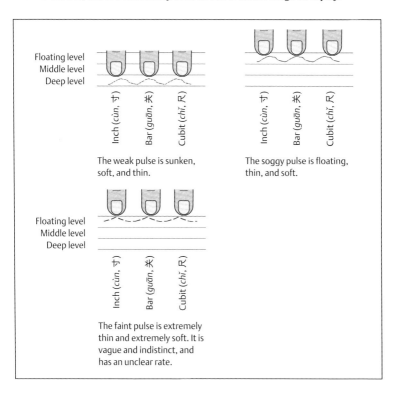

The weak pulse is sunken, soft, and thin.

The soggy pulse is floating, thin, and soft.

The faint pulse is extremely thin and extremely soft. It is vague and indistinct, and has an unclear rate.

▓ Indications

• The fine pulse indicates *qi* and blood vacuity, all types of vacuity, or taxation detriment (*láo sǔn*, 劳损). The fine pulse can also indicate damp evil accumulating and stagnating in the interior. When damp evil invades the body, encumbers the spleen and stomach, or lingers in the channels and network vessels, the pulse is fine.

▓ Concurrent Pulses and their Indications

Concurrent Pulse Manifestations	Manifesting Symptoms
Fine and stringlike	*Yin* vacuity of the liver and kidney
Fine and rapid	*Yin* vacuity or blood vacuity with heat
Fine and rough	Blood vacuity or blood stasis
Fine and faint	*Yang* vacuity with *yin* exuberance
Sunken and fine	Interior vacuity or damp impediment

The Intermittent Pulse (*Dài Mài*, 代脉)

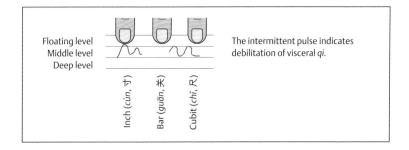

Floating level
Middle level
Deep level

Inch (*cùn*, 寸) Bar (*guān*, 关) Cubit (*chǐ*, 尺)

The intermittent pulse indicates debilitation of visceral *qi*.

▓ Pulse Manifestation

• The intermittent pulse pauses periodically at regular intervals.
• The intermittent pulse can be sluggish or hurried, depending on the disease condition.
• It pauses at regular intervals, each pause being of relatively long duration.

▨ Pulse Principles

- When *qi* and blood are depleted and there is debilitation of visceral *qi*, or there is wind damage, severe pain, fright and fear, or injury from external trauma, the pulse *qi* is unable to pulsate continuously, resulting in an intermittent pulse.
- If a pregnant woman exhibits an intermittent pulse, this is because the *qi* and blood are being used to nourish the fetus.

▨ Differentiation

The intermittent pulse is similar to the bound and skipping pulses. All three pulses are interrupted periodically.

▨ Comparing the Pulses

- The intermittent pulse is more sluggish than the skipping pulse. It pauses at regular intervals, each pause being of relatively long duration.
- The bound pulse is sluggish and skips a beat at irregular intervals. The duration of each pause is relatively short.
- The skipping pulse is urgent and rapid. It skips a beat at irregular intervals. The duration of each pause is relatively short.

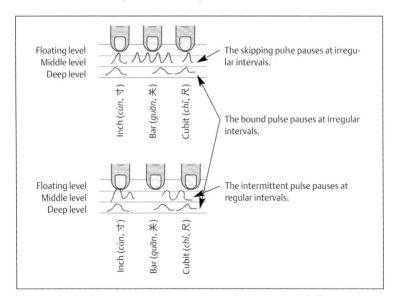

▥ Indications

- The intermittent pulse indicates the debilitation of visceral *qi*. For example, in cases of chronic diarrhea or chronic dysentery, which leads to a decline of spleen *qi*, the pulse is intermittent.
- Other conditions may occasionally also be accompanied by an intermittent pulse. These include wind damage, severe pain, fright and fear, and injury from external trauma.

▥ Concurrent Pulses and their Indications

Concurrent Pulse Manifestations	Manifesting Symptoms
Intermittent, moderate, and weak	Debilitation of visceral *qi*
Intermittent and rapid	Wind damage, severe pain, or fright and fear

The Short Pulse (*Duǎn Mài*, 短脉)

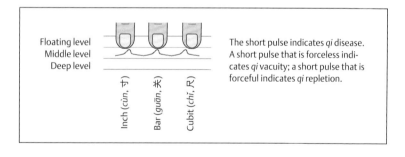

Floating level
Middle level
Deep level

Inch (*cùn*, 寸) Bar (*guān*, 关) Cubit (*chǐ*, 尺)

The short pulse indicates *qi* disease. A short pulse that is forceless indicates *qi* vacuity; a short pulse that is forceful indicates *qi* repletion.

▥ Pulse Manifestation

- The shape of the short pulse is short and small. It does not fill up the normal pulse positions.
- The short pulse is shorter and smaller than the normal pulse manifestation. The short pulse does not fill the boundaries of the normal pulse positions.

Pulse Principles

- A short, forceless pulse: When *yang qi* is depleted, there is insufficient force to propel the circulation of blood, thus giving rise to a short and forceless pulse.
- A short, forceful pulse: *Qi* stagnation, blood stasis, phlegm–rheum, or food accumulation leading to blockage of the pulse *qi* and its inability to ascend and expand, result in a short and forceful pulse.

Differentiation

The short pulse is similar to the stirred pulse. The shape of both pulses is short and small.

Comparing the Pulses

- The shape of the short pulse is short and small. It does not fill up the normal pulse positions.
- The stirred pulse is smooth and evasive like a bean. It is slippery, rapid, and forceful. It oscillates and is unstable.

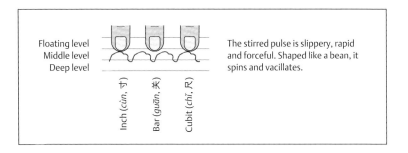

Floating level
Middle level
Deep level

Inch (*cùn*, 寸) Bar (*guān*, 关) Cubit (*chǐ*, 尺)

The stirred pulse is slippery, rapid and forceful. Shaped like a bean, it spins and vacillates.

Indications

- The short pulse indicates *qi* disease.
- A short pulse that is forceless indicates *qi* vacuity pattern, which includes signs and symptoms such as palpitations, spontaneous sweating, shortness of breath, laziness of speech, and fatigue of the body with lack of strength.
- A short pulse that is forceful indicates *qi* repletion pattern, such as symptoms caused by *qi* stagnation, blood stasis, phlegm–rheum, and food accumulation.

Concurrent Pulses and their Indications

Concurrent Pulse Manifestations	Manifesting Symptoms
Short and floating	Lung *qi* vacuity or inhibited blood flow
Short and rough	Heart *qi* vacuity or inhibited blood flow
Short and sunken	Glomus or stasis obstruction of the heart vessels
Short and slow	Vacuity cold

The Replete Pulse (*Shí Mài*, 實脈)

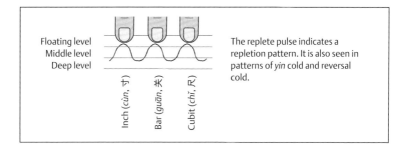

Floating level
Middle level
Deep level

Inch (*cùn*, 寸)   Bar (*guān*, 关)   Cubit (*chǐ*, 尺)

The replete pulse indicates a repletion pattern. It is also seen in patterns of *yin* cold and reversal cold.

Pulse Manifestation

- The pulse is forceful at all three levels (superficial, middle, and deep).
- The replete pulse is forceful regardless of the depth at which it is palpated. It feels substantial under the fingers. The pulse is large and powerfully strong.

Pulse Principles

- When there is exuberance of evil *qi* in the body without right qi vacuity, the evil *qi* and right *qi* will battle with each other, causing the *qi* and blood within the vessels to become congested. When the vessels become hardened and full, the pulse beat will be replete and forceful.

■ Differentiation

The replete pulse is similar to the tight, firm, and surging pulses. They are all relatively strong pulse manifestations.

■ Comparing the Pulses

- Although the replete pulse is not as vigorous as the surging pulse, it is forceful at both the superficial and deep levels, with an extremely strong onset and recession.
- The tight pulse is taut, tense, and forceful. It is like a twisted rope or cord.
- When palpated lightly, the surging pulse feels like a boat amidst the turbulence of great waves. It has a strong onset and a weak recession. When palpated deeply, it feels weak.

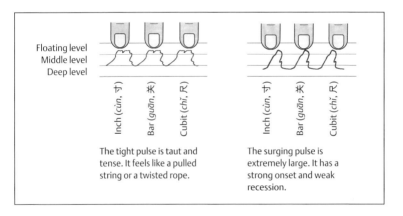

The tight pulse is taut and tense. It feels like a pulled string or a twisted rope.

The surging pulse is extremely large. It has a strong onset and weak recession.

■ Indications

- The replete pulse indicates a repletion pattern. Superabundance of exuberant fire and heat evils in the body manifesting as mania with delirious speech, congestion of the *qi* dynamic and constipation, inhibited flow of visceral and bowel *qi*, or exuberant triple burner fire can all give rise to a replete pulse.
- The replete pulse can also show up in cases of *yin* cold and reversal cold. Long-term *yin* cold and reversal cold leading to debilitation of *qi* and blood should be accompanied by a vacuous and faint pulse. However, in this case, the pulse is replete, which shows that the pulse and signs are contradictory, making this an unusual pulse manifestation.

- A person of normal health can also exhibit a replete pulse; this means that the right *qi* is abundant and that the viscera and bowels are functioning well.

▨ Concurrent Pulses and their Indications

Concurrent Pulse Manifestations	Manifesting Symptoms
Floating and replete	Repletion of exterior evil
Sunken and replete	Repletion of interior evil, distension and fullness, constipation, and accumulation and stagnation
Surging and replete	Repletion heat
Slippery and replete	Phlegm congealing

The Long Pulse (*Cháng Mài,* 長脈)

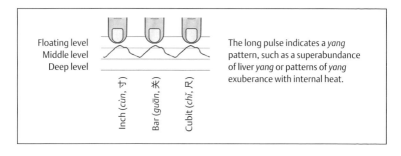

Floating level
Middle level
Deep level

Inch (*cùn,* 寸)
Bar (*guān,* 关)
Cubit (*chǐ,* 尺)

The long pulse indicates a *yang* pattern, such as a superabundance of liver *yang* or patterns of *yang* exuberance with internal heat.

▨ Pulse Manifestation

- The length of the long pulse exceeds the boundaries of the normal pulse positions.
- The long pulse is longer and straighter than the normal pulse manifestation. Its length far exceeds the boundaries of the usual inch, bar, and cubit pulse positions.

Pulse Principles

- The long pulse has two forms:
- A long pulse in a person of normal health shows that the pulse *qi* is unimpeded. The pulse manifestation is soft and moderate. This is known as the normal pulse (*ping mài*, 平脉).
- If there is a superabundance and exuberance of liver *yang*, or if there is internal heat from exuberant *yang*, there will be a struggle between evil *qi* and right *qi*. This will give rise to a long pulse, which manifests as long, straight, and unyielding.

Differentiation

The long pulse is similar to the stringlike pulse. Both types of pulse are exceptionally long and straight.

Comparing the Pulses

- The long pulse extends beyond the boundaries of the original pulse positions. Its length far exceeds that of the inch, bar, and cubit pulse positions.
- The stringlike pulse is like the string of a musical instrument that has been stretched tight. Although it lacks the round and slippery smoothness, it does not extend beyond the boundaries of the original pulse positions.

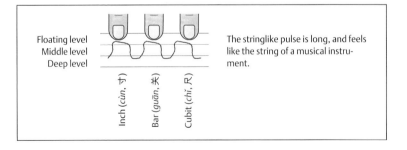

Floating level
Middle level
Deep level

Inch (*cùn*, 寸)   Bar (*guān*, 关)   Cubit (*chǐ*, 尺)

The stringlike pulse is long, and feels like the string of a musical instrument.

Indications

- The long pulse indicates a *yang* pattern, such as superabundance of liver *yang* or abnormally exuberant *yang* causing accumulation of internal heat.

Concurrent Pulses and their Indications

Concurrent Pulse Manifestations	Manifesting Symptoms
Long and stringlike	Liver disease
Long, surging, and forceful	Yang brightness heat exuberance
Long and replete	Evil *qi* binding internally
Long and slippery	Phlegm–heat congestion
Long, sunken, and fine	Accumulations and gatherings (*jī jù*, 積聚)

The Slippery Pulse (*Huá Mài*, 滑脈)

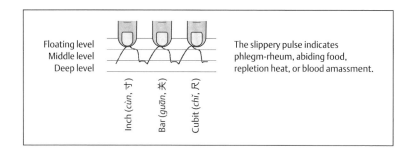

Floating level
Middle level
Deep level

Inch (*cùn*, 寸)
Bar (*guān*, 关)
Cubit (*chǐ*, 尺)

The slippery pulse indicates phlegm-rheum, abiding food, repletion heat, or blood amassment.

Pulse Manifestation

- The slippery pulse has a smooth onset and recession. It is smooth and evasive, like pearls rolling on a dish.
- The beating of the slippery pulse is smooth and evasive, like pearls. The beat is extremely fluid. It gives off a repeatedly rotating, smooth and evasive, and unhindered feeling.

Pulse Principles

- When there is evil *qi* congestion in the body, if the right *qi* is not weakened by the onslaught, the right *qi* and the evil *qi* will contend with each other, leading to the repletion and exuberance of the *qi* dynamic and causing the

blood to flow swiftly and surge. As a result, the pulse has an extremely fluid onset and recession, and feels smooth and evasive under the fingers.
- When a person of normal health exhibits a slippery pulse, it should be slippery and moderate. This is due to an abundance of *qi* and blood, and smooth and unimpeded blood circulation.
- If a pregnant woman exhibits a slippery pulse, this means that *qi* and blood are plentiful and harmonious.

Differentiation

The slippery pulse is similar to the rapid pulse. The rates of both pulse type are faster than normal.

Comparing the Pulses

- The onset and recession of the slippery pulse are extremely smooth. The shape of the pulse is smooth, evasive, and fluid, like a ball in repeated rotation.
- The rapid pulse beats more than five times per respiration.

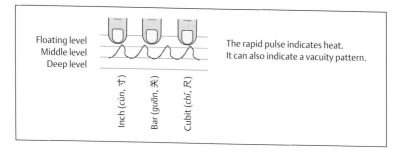

Floating level
Middle level
Deep level

Inch (*cùn*, 寸)　Bar (*guān*, 关)　Cubit (*chǐ*, 尺)

The rapid pulse indicates heat.
It can also indicate a vacuity pattern.

Indications

- The slippery pulse indicates phlegm-rheum, abiding food, repletion heat, or blood amassment (*xù xuè*, 蓄血).
- The pulse will manifest as slippery if there is phlegm–drool congestion in the lung causing panting, cough, *qi* counterflow, and phlegm rale; stagnation of abiding food leading to abdominal distention and bound stool; evil heat brewing internally, engendering heat effusion (fever) and heat reversal;

damp–heat pouring downward causing difficult painful urination; or blood amassment in the lower burner.

- A slippery pulse can also indicate a debilitation of original *qi*. When the *qi* and blood of the body are debilitated, the remaining *qi* and blood will linger between the viscera and bowels, and the channels and network vessels. This results in the manifestation of a slippery pulse, indicating the outward discharge of original *qi*.

▤ Concurrent Pulses and their Indications

Concurrent Pulse Manifestations	Manifesting Symptoms
Floating and slippery	Wind–phlegm
Sunken and slippery	Phlegm–food
Slippery and rapid	Phlegm–fire, damp–heat, or exuberant heat
Slippery and stringlike	Phlegm gathering

The Stringlike Pulse (*Xián Mài*, 弦脉)

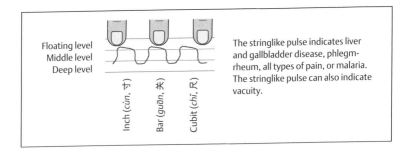

Floating level
Middle level
Deep level

Inch (*cùn*, 寸)   Bar (*guān*, 关)   Cubit (*chǐ*, 尺)

The stringlike pulse indicates liver and gallbladder disease, phlegm–rheum, all types of pain, or malaria. The stringlike pulse can also indicate vacuity.

▤ Pulse Manifestation

- The stringlike pulse is long, and feels like the string of a musical instrument.
- The stringlike pulse is straight and long. It is more taut and distended than normal. Using the string of a musical instrument as an example, the tension of the string is increased if the two ends are stretched tight. The stringlike

pulse is not limited to a certain rate or depth. It can occur simultaneously with the floating or sunken, and with the rapid or slow, pulse.

▧ Pulse Principles

- The stringlike pulse is a manifestation of the gathering and distention of the pulse *qi*.
- The main functions of the liver are to govern free coursing and to regulate the *qi* dynamic (which should be gentle and mild). If the liver's function of free coursing is impaired due to congestion of evil *qi* in the body, this will cause the *qi* dynamic to be obstructed as well. As a result, the pulse will be stringlike.
- If pain from interior static blood or phlegm–rheum congestion leads to obstruction in the *qi* dynamic, *yin* and *yang* will no longer be in harmony. As a result, the pulse will be tense and inhibited, giving rise to a stringlike pulse.

▧ Differentiation

The stringlike pulse is similar to the tight pulse. The pulse *qi* of both pulses are tense.

▧ Comparing the Pulses

- The stringlike pulse is long, and feels like pressing on the string of a musical instrument.
- The tight pulse feels like pressing on a string or rope that has been stretched and pulled tight. It is tense, taut, and forceful.

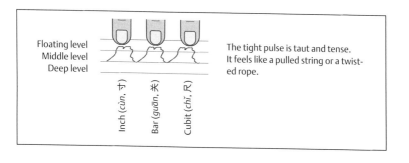

Floating level
Middle level
Deep level

Inch (*cùn*, 寸)   Bar (*guān*, 关)   Cubit (*chǐ*, 尺)

The tight pulse is taut and tense. It feels like a pulled string or a twisted rope.

▨ Indications

- The stringlike pulse indicates liver and gallbladder repletion. Symptoms include the counterflow ascent of *qi* dynamic affecting the head and face (causing veiling dizziness and headaches), chest and hypochondriac pain, or hypertonicity of the limbs.
- The stringlike pulse indicates phlegm–rheum. Symptoms include cough and counterflow with panting and fullness, palpitations, and shortness of breath.
- The stringlike pulse indicates all types of pain. Symptoms include distention in the stomach duct and abdomen that likes pressure, cold mounting pain, and impediment pain.
- The stringlike pulse indicates malaria. Symptoms include the alternating chills and fever induced by the onset of malaria, or lesser *yang* disease pattern.
- The stringlike pulse can also indicate a vacuity pattern. *Qi* and blood vacuity or insufficiency of original *qi* can also produce a stringlike pulse.

▨ Concurrent Pulses and their Indications

Concurrent Pulse Manifestations	Manifesting Symptoms
Stringlike and rapid	Liver and gallbladder repletion fire
Stringlike and slow	Vacuity cold
Stringlike and tight	All types of pain or mounting *qi*
Stringlike and fine	Hypertonicity
Floating and stringlike	Propping rheum and wind evil headache
Stringlike and slippery	Phlegm–rheum
Stringlike, large, and forceless	Vacuity pattern

The Tight Pulse (*Jǐn Mài*, 緊脈)

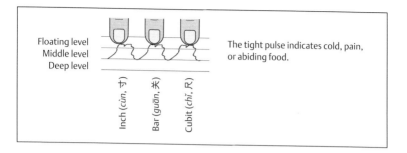

Floating level
Middle level
Deep level

Inch (*cùn*, 寸)
Bar (*guān*, 关)
Cubit (*chǐ*, 尺)

The tight pulse indicates cold, pain, or abiding food.

■ Pulse Manifestation

- The tight pulse is taut and tense. It feels like a pulled string or a twisted rope.
- The quality of the tight pulse is tense. It is forceful, and has the same twisted instability of a cord that has been pulled tight and flicked by the fingers.

■ Pulse Principles

- Since the nature of cold evil is to cause constriction and tautness as well as congealing and stagnation, when cold evil invades the body, it leads to the tight contraction and hypertonicity of the blood vessels. This results in a tight pulse, which feels tense and taut.

■ Differentiation

The tight pulse is similar to the stringlike pulse; both pulse manifestations are tense.

■ Comparing the Pulses

- The quality of the tight pulse is tense. It is forceful, and has the same twisted instability of a cord that has been pulled tight and flicked by the fingers.
- The stringlike pulse also has a taut and tense quality. Although it lacks the round slippery smoothness, it does not, unlike the tight pulse, feel finger-flicked or twisted.

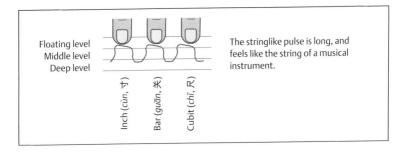

Floating level
Middle level
Deep level

Inch (cùn, 寸)   Bar (guān, 关)   Cubit (chǐ, 尺)

The stringlike pulse is long, and feels like the string of a musical instrument.

▦ **Indications**

- The tight pulse indicates a cold pattern.
- The tight pulse indicates pain (primarily cold-induced pain).
- The tight pulse indicates accumulation and stagnation of abiding food, such as retention of food in the abdomen with indigestion.

▦ **Concurrent Pulses and their Indications**

Concurrent Pulse Manifestations	Manifesting Symptoms
Floating and tight	Exterior cold repletion pattern
Sunken and tight	Interior cold or phlegm–rheum abiding food
Tight and stringlike	Pain or tetany

3 Analyses of the Pulse Manifestations and Signs of Common Diseases

Chinese medicine believes that the causes of all disease include the six excesses (wind, cold, summerheat, dampness, dryness, and fire), the seven affects (joy, anger, anxiety, thought, sorrow, fear, and fright), external injury, static blood, phlegm-rheum, food accumulation, and damage due to sexual intemperance. However, during the passage and transmutation of the disease, one must differentiate between exterior and interior, vacuity and repletion, and cold and heat. Therefore, even if different patients were to suffer the same disease pattern, they would not necessarily exhibit exactly the same pulse manifestation. It is imperative that beginners are aware of this when arriving at a clinical diagnosis.

For instance, let us take fever from external contraction as an example. Although we are talking about the same symptom (fever), if a patient of relatively weak constitution has a fever, this for the most part belongs to an exterior vacuity pattern, and the pulse manifestation is floating and moderate or floating and weak; if a patient of relatively strong constitution has a fever, this for the

The pulse manifestation of chronic hepatitis

Liver depression and *qi* stagnation (repletion pattern).

Cold–damp obstructing the center (vacuity–repletion complex pattern).

the disease condition shifts to

Stringlike pulse.

Sunken and stringlike pulse or sunken and slow pulse.

most part belongs to an exterior repletion pattern, and the pulse manifestation would be floating and tight, or floating and rapid.

Let us take as a further example chronic hepatitis. If a patient of relatively strong constitution suffers from chronic hepatitis, this would usually be considered to be a repletion pattern of liver depression and *qi* stagnation, and the pulse would be stringlike. However, if in the case of chronic hepatitis, the disease condition shifts to cold–damp obstructing the center (a vacuity–repletion complex pattern) because of a prolonged and lingering disease course that has led to *qi* and blood vacuity or caused damage to the original *yang* of the spleen and kidney, the pulse will manifest as sunken and stringlike, or sunken and slow.

The following table is a list of common disease patterns with their corresponding indications and pulse manifestations, which will be discussed later on in this chapter.

Head and Body Heat Effusion (Fever)

Pattern 1: Wind–Cold Exterior Vacuity
Signs and symptoms: Fever, aversion to cold, headache, aversion to wind after sweating, a pale tongue, white tongue fur, and a pulse that is floating and moderate, or floating and weak.
▶ See also page 103.

Pattern 2: Wind–Cold Exterior Repletion
Signs and symptoms: Fever, aversion to cold, absence of sweating, generalized body pain and bone pain, a pale tongue, white tongue fur, and a pulse that is floating and tight, or floating and rapid.
▶ See also page 104.

Pattern 3: Repletion Heat Binding Internally
Signs and symptoms: Glomus and fullness of the stomach duct and abdomen, constipation, tidal heat with delirious speech, a red tongue, dry and burnt-yellow tongue fur with prickles, and a pulse that is sunken, slow, and forceful.
▶ See also page 106.

Pattern 4: Liver Depression and Qi Stagnation
Signs and symptoms: Rib-side pain, alternating fever and aversion to cold, belching, deep sighing, distention and fullness in the stomach duct and abdomen, yellow tongue fur, and a stringlike pulse.
▶ See also page 107.

Head and Body Heat Effusion (Fever)

Pattern 5: Spleen Vacuity Water Retention
Signs and symptoms: Dizziness, panting and cough, palpitations, counterflow fullness below the heart, sloppy stool with torpid intake, a pale and enlarged tongue with pronounced tooth marks, white glossy, slimy tongue fur, and a pulse that is sunken and tight, or sunken and stringlike.
▶ See also page 109.

Pattern 6: Yang *Vacuity with Contraction of Cold*
Signs and symptoms: Fever, aversion to cold, absence of sweating, headache, pain in the limbs and body, a pale tongue, white tongue fur, and a sunken and weak pulse.
▶ See also page 111.

Cough

Pattern 1: Phlegm–Heat Congestion in the Lung
Signs and symptoms: Cough, panting, and cough with rough breathing, thick sticky yellow phlegm, fever or absence of fever, a slightly red tongue body, yellow or yellow and slightly dry tongue fur, and a slippery and rapid pulse.
▶ See also page 112.

Pattern 2: Spleen Vacuity Water Retention
Signs and symptoms: Dizziness, panting and cough, palpitations, counterflow fullness below the heart, sloppy stool with torpid intake, a pale and enlarged tongue with pronounced tooth marks, white glossy, slimy tongue fur, and a pulse that is sunken and tight, or sunken and stringlike.
▶ See also page 113.

Pattern 3: Dampness Evil Obstructing the Lung
Signs and symptoms: Headache and dizzy vision, cough and hasty panting, pain in the chest and back, dry retching, a pale tongue with white slimy tongue fur, and a sunken and tight pulse.
▶ See also page 115.

Bronchitis

Pattern 1: Phlegm–Heat Congestion in the Lung
Signs and symptoms: Somber facial complexion, dark purple lips, chest pain and panting, a severe cough with an inability to lie flat, thick sticky yellow or white phlegm, a red tongue body with yellow tongue fur, and a slippery and rapid pulse.
▶ See also page 116.

Bronchitis

Pattern 2: Liver Depression and Qi Stagnation

Signs and symptoms: Bitter fullness in the chest and rib-side, vexation with rashness and irascibility, dizziness and tinnitus, dry mouth, dry stool, short voidings of reddish urine, a red tongue with yellow tongue fur, and a rapid and stringlike pulse.

▶ See also page 117.

Pattern 3: Cold–Rheum Obstructing the Lung

Signs and symptoms: Headache, severe cough and panting with an inability to lie flat that is mild during the day and worse at night, chest oppression, palpitations, copious thin white phlegm, a pale tongue with white or glossy slimy tongue fur, and a pulse that is floating and slippery, or sunken and tight.

▶ See also page 119.

High Blood Pressure

Pattern 1: Exuberant Internal Vacuity Cold, Counterflow Ascent of Phlegm Turbidity

Signs and symptoms: Headache (worse at the vertex), vexation and agitation, reversal cold of the extremities, dry retching or ejection of foamy drool, a pale enlarged tongue with tooth marks, white glossy slimy tongue fur, and a pulse that is sunken and stringlike, or sunken and slow.

▶ See also page 121.

Pattern 2: Liver Depression and Gallbladder Stagnation, Disharmony of the Qi Dynamic

Signs and symptoms: Bitter fullness in the chest and rib-side, vexation with rashness and irascibility, dizziness and tinnitus, a dry mouth, dry stools, short voidings of reddish urine, a red tongue with yellow tongue fur, and a rapid and stringlike pulse.

▶ See also page 123.

Heart Disease

Pattern 1: Water Qi Intimidating the Heart (Vacuity–Repletion Complex)

Signs and symptoms: Oppression and dull pain in the chest or severe pain in the chest and back, palpitations, dizzy vision, a pale enlarged tongue body with pronounced tooth marks, white moist tongue fur, and a pulse that is sunken and tight, or stringlike.

▶ See also page 124.

Heart Disease

Pattern 2: Debilitation of Kidney Yang, Cold Water Flooding Upward
Signs and symptoms: Dizziness, palpitations, chest pain radiating through to the back, physical cold and cold limbs, a pale moist tongue with white glossy tongue fur, and a pulse that is sunken and faint, or bound and intermittent.
▶ See also page 126.

Pattern 3: Phlegm and Heat Binding Together, Obstruction of Heart Yang
Signs and symptoms: Glomus and fullness of the chest and stomach duct, phlegm rale, palpitations, constipation, a red-tipped tongue, yellow and slimy tongue fur, and a pulse that is slippery and stringlike, or rapid and stringlike.
▶ See also page 128.

Pattern 4: Insufficiency of Qi and Blood, Dual Vacuity of Yin and Yang
Signs and symptoms: Chest oppression and pain, palpitations, a shortage of *qi* and lack of strength, a pale tongue with moist white tongue fur, and a bound and intermittent pulse.
▶ See also page 129.

Gastric Ulcer

Pattern 1: Liver and Stomach Yin Vacuity
Signs and symptoms: Dry mouth and throat, distending pain in the stomach duct, hypertonicity and pain of the four limbs, dry bound stools, a red and tender tongue tip that is lacking in moisture, and a fine, stringlike pulse.
▶ See also page 131.

Pattern 2: Spleen–Stomach Vacuity Cold
Signs and symptoms: Glomus, fullness, and distending pain of the chest and stomach duct that likes pressure and warmth; upwelling and vomiting of clear water; a bland taste in the mouth with torpid intake (*nà dāi*, 納呆); lack of warmth in the extremities; sloppy, rotten stools; a pale, enlarged, tooth-marked tongue with white, moist, and slightly slimy tongue fur; and a moderate, weak pulse.
▶ See also page 132.

Gastric Ulcer

Pattern 3: Cold–Heat Complex (Vacuity–Repletion Complex)

Signs and symptoms: Vomiting, glomus and fullness or distending pain in the stomach duct, clamoring stomach (*cáo zá*, 嘈雜), acid upflow, hunger with no desire to eat, rumbling intestines and diarrhea, a pale and enlarged tongue with slimy, yellow (or white) tongue fur, and a pulse that is (a) sunken, (b) fine and weak, or (c) fine and stringlike.

▶ See also page 134.

Liver Cirrhosis

Pattern 1: Liver Depression and Damp Obstruction (Vacuity–Repletion Complex)

Signs and symptoms: Dizzy head and vision, vexation with rashness and irascibility, rib-side pain, glomus and fullness of the chest and diaphragm, reduced food intake, distention after meals, short voidings of reddish urine, white glossy tongue fur, and a stringlike pulse.

▶ See also page 136.

Pattern 2: Damp–Heat Brewing Internally

Signs and symptoms: Nausea and vomiting, fever and thirst, yellowing of the body and eyes (resembling the color of a tangerine), distention and fullness in the abdomen, scanty yellow urine, constipation, a red tongue tip and margins, yellow slimy tongue fur, and a pulse that is rapid, slippery, and stringlike.

▶ See also page 137.

Pattern 3: Water–Rheum Collecting and Binding

Signs and symptoms: Oppression and pain in the chest and rib-side, an enlarged abdomen with glomus and fullness, abdominal distention that is worse after meals, nausea and vomiting, shortness of breath, short voidings of reddish urine, white glossy tongue fur, and a pulse that is sunken and stringlike.

▶ See also page 139.

Chronic Hepatitis

Pattern 1: Liver Depression and Qi Stagnation

Signs and symptoms: Bitter taste in the mouth, rib-side distention and pain, hepatomegaly, glomus of the stomach duct, abdominal distention, white and yellow tongue fur, and a stringlike pulse.

▶ See also page 140.

Chronic Hepatitis

Pattern 2: Cold–Damp Obstructing the Center (Vacuity–Repletion Complex)

Signs and symptoms: Dark and gloomy yellowing of the body that resembles the color of smoke, reduced food intake with oppression in the stomach duct, fear of cold and cold limbs, sloppy diarrhea, yellow urine, a pale tongue with white glossy tongue fur, and a pulse that is sunken and stringlike, or sunken and slow.

▶ See also page 142.

Diabetes

Pattern 1: Intense Stomach Heat

Signs and symptoms: Great thirst with fluid intake, increased eating with rapid hungering, sweating, short voidings of reddish urine, vexation, a red tongue with dry yellow tongue fur, and a pulse that is surging and large, or slippery and rapid.

▶ See also page 144.

Pattern 2: Yin Humor Depletion

Signs and symptoms: Thirst with increased fluid intake, a dry throat, vexation and agitation, pain and hypertonicity of the limbs, dry stools, short voidings of scant urine, a dry red tongue with scant tongue fur, and a pulse that is stringlike and fine, or rapid, fine and forceless.

▶ See also page 145.

Pattern 3: Binding of Dampness and Heat (Vacuity–Repletion Complex)

Signs and symptoms: Thirst with increased fluid intake, increased eating with rapid hungering, vexation and insomnia, inhibited urination, diarrhea, a red tongue with scanty or no tongue fur, and a pulse that is floating and rapid, or fine and rapid.

▶ See also page 147.

Pattern 4: Interior Heat Binding and Gathering

Signs and symptoms: Vexation and thirst with an increased intake of fluids; a dry mouth and tongue; increased eating with rapid hungering; tidal fever with sweating; fullness, distention, and pain of the abdomen; constipation; short voidings of reddish urine; a red tongue with dry yellow tongue fur or prickles; and a pulse that is slippery and rapid, or sunken, replete, and forceful.

▶ See also page 148.

Diabetes

Pattern 5: Blood Stasis and Stomach Heat
Signs and symptoms: Thirst without an increased intake of fluids, fatigue, paralysis of the four limbs, constipation with hard or bound stools, a dark purple tongue with thin yellow or white tongue fur, and a pulse that is stringlike and slippery, or sunken and fine.
▶ See also page 150.

Chronic Nephritis

Pattern 1: Kidney Vacuity with Damp Depression, and Binding of Water and Heat (Vacuity–Repletion Complex)
Signs and symptoms: Dizziness and tinnitus, limp, aching lumbus and knees, puffy face and swelling of the feet, frequent but incomplete urination that is worse at night, low-grade fever, vexing heat in the five centers, a red tongue with scant tongue fur or a pale tongue with white tongue fur, and a pulse that is stringlike, fine, and rapid.
▶ See also page 152.

Pattern 2: Lower Burner Damp–Heat and Water Amassment in the Bladder
Signs and symptoms: Thirst, fever, fear of cold, urinary frequency, urinary urgency, painful or incessant dribbling urination, distending pain in the lesser abdomen, aching pain in the lumbus, thin yellow tongue fur, and a pulse that is soggy and rapid, or slippery and rapid.
▶ See also page 154.

Sciatica

Pattern 1: Enduring Impediment Entering the Network Vessels
Signs and symptoms: Prolonged pain in the lumbus and legs, gradual emaciation of the flesh with numbness and inhibited bending and stretching, difficult mobility, cold and fatigued limbs, a pale tongue with thin white tongue fur, and a fine, weak pulse.
▶ See also page 156.

Pattern 2: Water–Damp Invasion
Signs and symptoms: Stiffness and pain in the lumbus and legs with inhibited bending and stretching, pain upon exposure to cold that is relieved by heat, thin white tongue fur, and a moderate, stringlike pulse.
▶ See also page 157.

Sciatica

Pattern 3: Congealing Phlegm–Damp
Signs and symptoms: Lumbar pain of fixed location that is worse at night, numbness, heavy and cumbersome lumbus and legs, thick slimy tongue fur, and a pulse that is slow and rough, or slippery.

▶ See also page 158.

Dysmenorrhea

Pattern 1: Liver Depression and Qi Stagnation
Signs and symptoms: Distending pain in the lower abdomen before or during menstruation; scant menstrual flow or inhibited menstruation; distention and oppression in the chest and rib-side; frequent sighing; premenstrual vexation, agitation, and irascibility; breast distention; a dull and stagnant-looking tongue with white tongue fur, and a stringlike pulse.

▶ See also page 160.

Pattern 2: Internal Static Blood Obstruction
Signs and symptoms: Premenstrual or menstrual lower abdominal hardness and pain that refuses pressure, dark purple menstrual flow with stasis clots, pain relief after passage of the clots, a soot-black facial complexion, encrusted skin (in severe cases), a purplish green-blue tongue with stasis macules, dark distended sublingual veins, thin white tongue fur, and a pulse that is sunken and rough, or sunken and bound.

▶ See also page 161.

Pattern 3: Blood Vacuity and Congealing Cold
Signs and symptoms: Premenstrual or menstrual lower abdominal pain that likes warmth and pressure, scant pale-colored menstrual flow, pain that is accompanied by cold or numb hands and feet, a pale tongue with white tongue fur, and a sunken, fine, and slow pulse.

▶ See also page 163.

Leukorrhea

Pattern 1: Yang Vacuity with Exuberant Dampness
Signs and symptoms: An incessant dribbling of thin white vaginal discharge that increases in quantity with exposure to cold, excruciating pain in the lumbus, cold pain in the lower abdomen, frequent long voidings of clear urine, sloppy diarrhea, a pale tongue with white, moist or glossy tongue fur, and a pulse that is sunken, slow, and weak.

▶ See also page 165.

Leukorrhea

Pattern 2: Exuberant Internal Damp–Heat

Signs and symptoms: A sticky, slimy, fishy-smelling vaginal discharge that is a yellow or yellow and white in color, chest oppression, a slimy sensation in the mouth, torpid intake, continuous dull pain in the lower abdomen, short voidings of reddish urine, a red tongue with yellow slimy tongue fur, and a soggy and rapid pulse.

▶ See also page 167.

Menopausal Syndrome

Pattern 1: Yin and Yang Vacuity Detriment

Signs and symptoms: Perimenopausal fever and sweating, dizziness and tinnitus, vexation and agitation, insomnia, a limp, aching lumbus and knees, cold limbs, thin white tongue fur, and a sunken, fine pulse.

▶ See also page 168.

Pattern 2: Liver and Kidney Yin Vacuity

Signs and symptoms: Perimenopausal limp, aching lumbus and knees, afternoon tidal fever, heat in the palms and soles, fullness and oppression in the chest and rib-side, vexation and agitation, insomnia, a bitter taste in the mouth, a dry throat, irregular menstruation, scant and thin menstrual flow, a red tongue, scant tongue fur, and a pulse that is stringlike, fine, and rapid.

▶ See also page 170.

■ Head and Body Heat Effusion (Fever)

Wind–Cold Exterior Vacuity

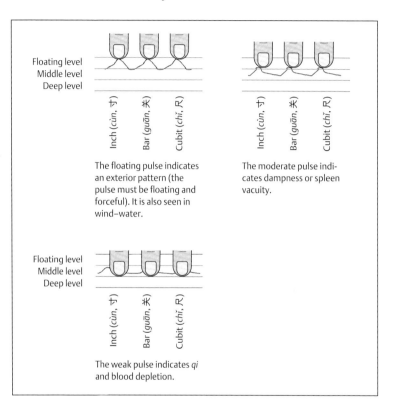

The floating pulse indicates an exterior pattern (the pulse must be floating and forceful). It is also seen in wind–water.

The moderate pulse indicates dampness or spleen vacuity.

The weak pulse indicates *qi* and blood depletion.

Signs and symptoms

Fever, aversion to cold, headache, aversion to wind after sweating, a pale tongue, white tongue fur, and a pulse that is floating and moderate, or floating and weak.

Fever:
The defense *qi* and evil *qi* fight with each other inside the body. The evil *qi* looks for an exit route but there is none, so it transforms into heat evil.

Aversion to cold:
Cold evil invades the fleshy exterior and impairs the defense *qi*'s function of warming the fleshy exterior.

Headache:
When the channels of the head are subjected to the invasion of cold evil, this gives rise to *qi* and blood stasis obstruction. When there is obstruction of *qi* and blood, there is pain.

Aversion to wind after sweating:
When the body sweats, the defense *qi* also seeps out of the body with the sweat. The defense *qi* can no longer warm the fleshy exterior, thus resulting in aversion to wind.

Pulse:
A floating and moderate, or a floating and weak pulse.

Analysis

- The floating pulse is felt with light palpation. Although its strength is slightly reduced when heavy pressure is applied, it does not feel empty.
- The moderate pulse is slightly faster than the slow pulse. It beats four times per respiration, and its arrival is leisurely.
- The weak pulse is felt at the deep level. It is soft and forceless.

Wind–Cold Exterior Repletion

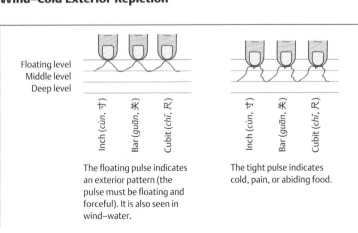

Floating level
Middle level
Deep level

Inch (*cùn*, 寸)   Bar (*guān*, 关)   Cubit (*chǐ*, 尺)

Inch (*cùn*, 寸)   Bar (*guān*, 关)   Cubit (*chǐ*, 尺)

The floating pulse indicates an exterior pattern (the pulse must be floating and forceful). It is also seen in wind–water.

The tight pulse indicates cold, pain, or abiding food.

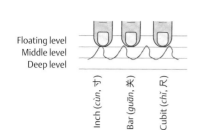

Floating level
Middle level
Deep level

Inch (*cùn*, 寸)
Bar (*guān*, 关)
Cubit (*chǐ*, 尺)

The rapid pulse indicates heat. The rapid pulse can also indicate a vacuity pattern.

Signs and symptoms

Fever, aversion to cold, absence of sweating, generalized body pain and bone pain, a pale tongue, white tongue fur, and a pulse that is floating and tight, or floating and rapid.

Fever:
The defense *qi* and evil *qi* fight with each other inside the body. The evil *qi* looks for an exit route but there is none, so it transforms into heat evil.

Aversion to cold:
Cold evil invades the fleshy exterior and impairs the defense *qi*'s function of warming the fleshy exterior.

Absence of sweating:
When wind–cold evil fetters the fleshy exterior, the normal diffusion of the *qi* dynamic is disrupted and the interstices are blocked, making it difficult for the sweat to be released. This leads to absence of sweating.

Headache:
When the channels of the head are subjected to the invasion of cold evil, this gives rise to *qi* and blood stasis obstruction. When there is obstruction of *qi* and blood, there is pain.

Generalized body pain and bone pain:
The channels of the entire body are subjected to the invasion of cold evil, leading to the obstruction and blockage of *qi* and blood. When there is obstruction of *qi* and blood, there is generalized body pain and bone pain.

Pulse:
A pulse that is floating and tight, or floating and rapid.

Analysis

- The floating pulse is felt with light palpation. Although its strength is slightly reduced when heavy pressure is applied, it does not feel empty.
- The tight pulse is taut and tense. It feels like a pulled string or a twisted rope.
- The rapid pulse beats five or more times per respiration.

Repletion Heat Binding Internally

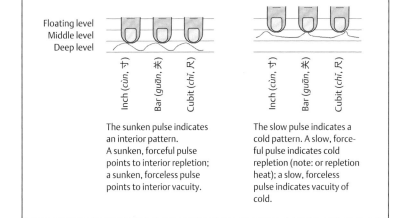

Floating level
Middle level
Deep level

Inch (cùn, 寸)   Bar (guān, 夫)   Cubit (chǐ, 尺)

Inch (cùn, 寸)   Bar (guān, 夫)   Cubit (chǐ, 尺)

The sunken pulse indicates an interior pattern. A sunken, forceful pulse points to interior repletion; a sunken, forceless pulse points to interior vacuity.

The slow pulse indicates a cold pattern. A slow, forceful pulse indicates cold repletion (note: or repletion heat); a slow, forceless pulse indicates vacuity of cold.

Signs and symptoms

Glomus and fullness of the stomach duct and abdomen, constipation, tidal heat with delirious speech, a red tongue, dry and burnt-yellow tongue fur with prickles, and a pulse that is sunken, slow, and forceful.

Glomus and fullness of the stomach duct and abdomen:
Phlegm turbidity or food accumulation becomes congested in the stomach and intestines, hindering the upbearing and downbearing of the *qi* dynamic of the stomach and intestines. As a result, there is glomus and fullness of the stomach duct and abdomen.

Constipation:
Due to long-term stasis and difficult digestion, phlegm turbidity or food accumulation can transform into heat. Heat

evil obstructing the intestinal tract has a tendency to disrupt the intestinal *qi* dynamic. If the heat is severe, it can also scorch and damage the fluids in the intestinal tract, impairing conveyance within the intestinal tract, and thus producing constipation.

Tidal heat with delirious speech:
Long-term accumulation, stagnation, and depression in the body transforms into heat. During the struggle between right *qi* and heat evil, damage to the *yin* humor by the heat evil will lead to depletion of *yin* humor. Heat evil will have no *yin* humor to attach itself to, and will transform into tidal heat. If the heat evil becomes congested in the heart chamber and harasses the heart spirit, this produces delirious speech.

Analysis

- The sunken pulse cannot be felt with light finger pressure. It is felt when heavy pressure is applied.
- The slow pulse has a slow onset and recession. It beats three times per respiration.

Liver Depression and *Qi* Stagnation

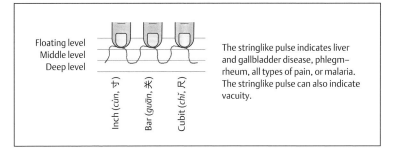

Floating level
Middle level
Deep level

Inch (*cùn*, 寸)   Bar (*guān*, 关)   Cubit (*chǐ*, 尺)

The stringlike pulse indicates liver and gallbladder disease, phlegm–rheum, all types of pain, or malaria. The stringlike pulse can also indicate vacuity.

Signs and symptoms

Rib-side pain, alternating fever and aversion to cold, belching, deep sighing, distention and fullness in the stomach duct and abdomen, yellow tongue fur, and a stringlike pulse.

Rib-side pain:
The liver channel passes through the chest and rib-side regions. When the *qi* and blood of the channel are obstructed, liver *qi* cannot flow smoothly, thus resulting in rib-side pain.

**Distention and fullness
in the stomach duct and abdomen:**
The liver channel passes through the lesser abdominal region. When the *qi* and blood of the liver channel are obstructed, the *qi* dynamic of the stomach duct and abdomen cannot flow smoothly, and this gives rise to distention and fullness in the stomach duct and abdomen.

Alternating fever and aversion to cold:
This is commonly a symptom belonging to lesser *yang* disease, emerging during the struggle between right and evil. During the onset of this symptom, when the patient is experiencing aversion to cold, there is no fever. When the patient has a fever, there is no aversion to cold. The alternating fever and aversion to cold may or may not occur at regular intervals.

Belching:
When there is obstruction of the *qi* dynamic due to liver–stomach disharmony, binding depression of liver *qi*, or food accumulation, this causes a sensation in the stomach that is similar to an upward surge of *qi*, accompanied by sounds. However, this symptom is different from frequent hiccoughs.

Deep sighing:
When there is obstruction of the *qi* dynamic due to failure of the lung *qi* to diffuse or binding depression of liver *qi*, this will manifest as frequent sighing.

Analysis

• The stringlike pulse is long, and feels like the string of a musical instrument.

Spleen Vacuity Water Retention

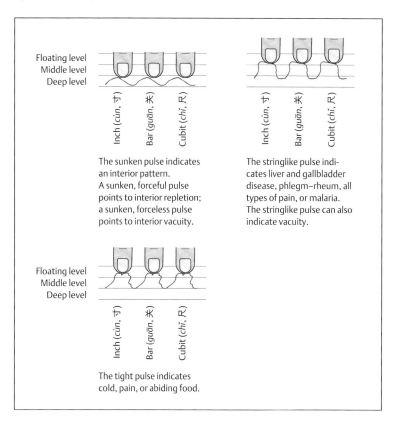

Floating level
Middle level
Deep level

Inch (cùn, 寸)
Bar (guān, 关)
Cubit (chǐ, 尺)

The sunken pulse indicates an interior pattern. A sunken, forceful pulse points to interior repletion; a sunken, forceless pulse points to interior vacuity.

Inch (cùn, 寸)
Bar (guān, 关)
Cubit (chǐ, 尺)

The stringlike pulse indicates liver and gallbladder disease, phlegm–rheum, all types of pain, or malaria. The stringlike pulse can also indicate vacuity.

Floating level
Middle level
Deep level

Inch (cùn, 寸)
Bar (guān, 关)
Cubit (chǐ, 尺)

The tight pulse indicates cold, pain, or abiding food.

Signs and symptoms

Dizziness, panting and cough, palpitations, counterflow fullness below the heart, sloppy stool with torpid take, a pale and enlarged tongue with pronounced tooth marks, white glossy, slimy tongue fur, and a pulse that is sunken and tight, or sunken and stringlike.

Dizziness:

Water–rheum or dampness evil clouds and blocks the head, eyes, and clear orifices, and prevents the clear *yang qi* from ascending and descending. This results in dizziness.

Panting and cough:

Phlegm turbidity moves with the upbearing and downbearing of the *qi* dynamic; it wants to exit the body, but cannot. This gives rise to panting and cough.

Palpitations:

Water–rheum or dampness evil invades the heart, obstructing the normal flow of *qi* and blood. This causes palpitations.

Counterflow fullness below the heart:

When water–rheum stagnates at the opening of the stomach and hinders the upbearing and downbearing of the stomach's *qi* dynamic, there will be a counterflow ascent of stomach *qi*. This results in counterflow fullness below the heart.

Sloppy stool with torpid intake:

When the spleen *qi* is vacuous, it is unable to transport and transform water–damp normally, causing it to collect in the stomach. This leads to abdominal fullness and a torpid intake of food. If water–damp pours downward into the intestinal tract, there will be sloppy diarrhea.

Pulse:

A pulse that is sunken and tight, or sunken and stringlike.

Analysis

- The sunken pulse cannot be felt with light finger pressure. It is felt when heavy pressure is applied.
- The tight pulse is taut and tense. It feels like a pulled string or a twisted rope.
- The stringlike pulse is long, and feels like the string of a musical instrument.

Yang **Vacuity with Contraction of Cold**

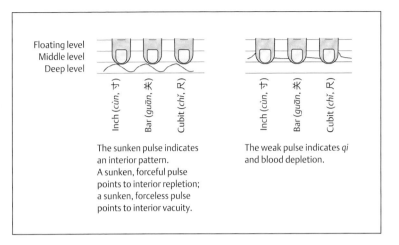

Floating level
Middle level
Deep level

Inch (cùn, 寸) Bar (guān, 关) Cubit (chǐ, 尺)

Inch (cùn, 寸) Bar (guān, 关) Cubit (chǐ, 尺)

The sunken pulse indicates an interior pattern.
A sunken, forceful pulse points to interior repletion; a sunken, forceless pulse points to interior vacuity.

The weak pulse indicates *qi* and blood depletion.

Signs and symptoms:

Fever, aversion to cold, absence of sweating, headache, pain in the limbs and body, a pale tongue, white tongue fur, and a sunken and weak pulse.

Fever:
The defense *qi* and evil *qi* fight each other inside the body. The evil *qi* looks for an exit route but there is none, so it transforms into heat evil.

Absence of sweating:
When wind–cold evil fetters the fleshy exterior, the normal diffusion of the *qi* dynamic is disrupted and the interstices are blocked, making it difficult for sweat to be released. This leads to an absence of sweating.

Aversion to cold:
Cold evil invades the fleshy exterior and

impairs the defense *qi*'s function of warming the fleshy exterior.

Headache:
When the channels of the head are subjected to the invasion of cold evil, this gives rise to *qi* and blood stasis obstruction. When there is obstruction of *qi* and blood, there is pain.

Pain in the limbs and body:
Cold evil fetters the four limbs and the fleshy exterior, obstructing the channels and the flow of *qi* and blood. This causes stasis obstruction in the channels; when there is obstruction, there is pain.

Analysis

- The sunken pulse cannot be felt with light finger pressure. It is felt when heavy pressure is applied.
- The weak pulse is felt at the deep level. It is soft and forceless.

■ Cough

Phlegm–Heat Congestion in the Lung

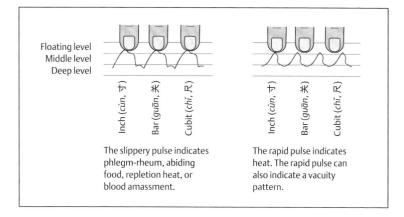

Floating level
Middle level
Deep level

Inch (*cùn*, 寸)   Bar (*guān*, 关)   Cubit (*chǐ*, 尺)

Inch (*cùn*, 寸)   Bar (*guān*, 关)   Cubit (*chǐ*, 尺)

The slippery pulse indicates phlegm-rheum, abiding food, repletion heat, or blood amassment.

The rapid pulse indicates heat. The rapid pulse can also indicate a vacuity pattern.

Signs and symptoms

Cough, panting and cough with rough breathing, thick sticky yellow phlegm, fever or absence of fever, a slightly red tongue body, yellow or yellow and slightly dry tongue fur, and a slippery and rapid pulse.

Cough:

Phlegm turbidity and evil heat congests the lung and obstructs the normal up-bearing and downbearing of the *qi* dynamic, resulting in cough.

Panting and cough with rough breathing:

Phlegm turbidity moves with the upbearing and downbearing of the *qi* dynamic; it wants to exit the body, but cannot. This will cause panting and cough with rough breathing.

Thick, sticky yellow phlegm:
Evil heat scorches and damages the body fluids. When the body fluids are depleted, there is thick, sticky yellow phlegm.

Fever or absence of fever:
During the struggle between evil heat and defense *qi*, there is fever if evil heat is able to penetrate outward into the fleshy exterior; if the interstices are tightly blocked, it is difficult for evil heat to penetrate outward into the fleshy exterior, in which case there is no fever.

Pulse:
A slippery and rapid pulse.

Analysis

- The slippery pulse has a smooth onset and recession. It is smooth and evasive, like pearls rolling on a dish.
- The rapid pulse beats five or more times per respiration.

Spleen Vacuity Water Retention

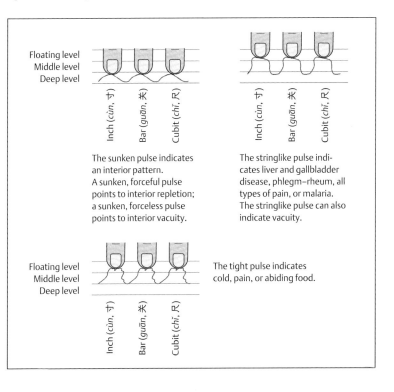

Floating level
Middle level
Deep level

Inch (cùn, 寸)   Bar (guān, 关)   Cubit (chǐ, 尺)

The sunken pulse indicates an interior pattern.
A sunken, forceful pulse points to interior repletion; a sunken, forceless pulse points to interior vacuity.

Inch (cùn, 寸)   Bar (guān, 关)   Cubit (chǐ, 尺)

The stringlike pulse indicates liver and gallbladder disease, phlegm–rheum, all types of pain, or malaria. The stringlike pulse can also indicate vacuity.

Floating level
Middle level
Deep level

Inch (cùn, 寸)   Bar (guān, 关)   Cubit (chǐ, 尺)

The tight pulse indicates cold, pain, or abiding food.

Signs and symptoms

Dizziness, panting and cough, palpitations, counterflow fullness below the heart, sloppy stool with torpid intake, a pale and enlarged tongue with pronounced tooth marks, white glossy, slimy tongue fur, and a pulse that is sunken and tight, or sunken and stringlike.

Dizziness:
Water–rheum or dampness evil clouds and blocks the head, eyes, and clear orifices, and prevents the clear *yang qi* from ascending and descending. This results in dizziness.

Panting and cough:
Phlegm turbidity moves with the upbearing and downbearing of the *qi* dynamic; it wants to exit the body, but cannot. This results in panting and cough.

Palpitations:
Water–rheum or dampness evil invades the heart, obstructing the normal flow of *qi* and blood. This causes palpitations.

Counterflow fullness below the heart:
The refers to the symptom caused by water–rheum collecting in the middle burner, which manifests as glomus, oppression, distention and fullness of the stomach duct, and counterflow ascent of stomach *qi*.

Sloppy stool:
This is caused by spleen *qi* vacuity detriment or insufficiency of kidney *yang*. The stool is clear, thin, grimy, and foul.

Torpid intake:
Also called "torpid stomach." The major cause of this is dullness of the stomach's ability to absorb nutrients and downbear turbidity.

Pulse:
A pulse that is sunken and tight, or sunken and stringlike.

Analysis

- The sunken pulse cannot be felt with light finger pressure. It is felt when heavy pressure is applied.
- The tight pulse is taut and tense. It feels like a pulled string or a twisted rope.
- The stringlike pulse is long, and feels like the string of a musical instrument.

Dampness Evil Obstructing the Lung

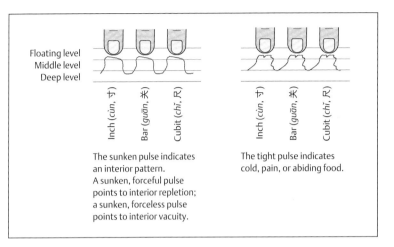

Floating level
Middle level
Deep level

Inch (*cùn*, 寸) Bar (*guān*, 关) Cubit (*chǐ*, 尺)

The sunken pulse indicates an interior pattern. A sunken, forceful pulse points to interior repletion; a sunken, forceless pulse points to interior vacuity.

Inch (*cùn*, 寸) Bar (*guān*, 关) Cubit (*chǐ*, 尺)

The tight pulse indicates cold, pain, or abiding food.

Signs and symptoms

Headache and dizzy vision, cough and hasty panting, pain in the chest and back, dry retching, a pale tongue with white slimy tongue fur, and a sunken and tight pulse.

Headache and dizzy vision:
Water–rheum or dampness evil clouds and blocks the head, eyes, and clear orifices, and prevents the clear *yang qi* from ascending and descending. This results in dizzy vision and headache.

Cough and hasty panting:
Dampness evil congests the lung and obstructs the normal upbearing and downbearing of the *qi* dynamic, resulting in cough and hasty panting.

Pain in the chest and back:
Water–rheum collecting and stagnating in the chest and back obstructs the flow of *qi* and blood in the channels and network vessels, producing pain in the chest and back.

Dry retching:
Water–rheum collecting and stagnating in the stomach disrupts the spleen and stomach's function of upbearing the clear and downbearing the turbid, leading to a counterflow ascent of stomach *qi*. This results in dry retching.

Pulse:
A sunken and tight pulse.

Analysis

- The sunken pulse cannot be felt with light finger pressure. It is felt when heavy pressure is applied.
- The tight pulse is taut and tense. It feels like a pulled string or a twisted rope.

■ Bronchitis

Phlegm–Heat Congestion in the Lung

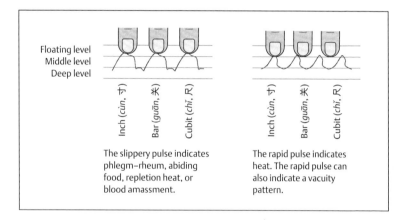

Floating level
Middle level
Deep level

Inch (cùn, 寸) Bar (guān, 关) Cubit (chǐ, 尺)

The slippery pulse indicates phlegm–rheum, abiding food, repletion heat, or blood amassment.

Inch (cùn, 寸) Bar (guān, 关) Cubit (chǐ, 尺)

The rapid pulse indicates heat. The rapid pulse can also indicate a vacuity pattern.

Signs and symptoms

A somber facial complexion, dark purple lips, chest pain and panting, severe cough with an inability to lie flat, thick sticky yellow or white phlegm, a red tongue body with yellow tongue fur, and a slippery and rapid pulse.

Recurrent cough with inability to lie flat:

Phlegm turbidity and evil heat congesting in the lung interfere with the normal depurative downbearing of lung qi, thus producing cough.

Chest pain and panting:

Phlegm turbidity collecting in the chest and diaphragm disrupts the flow of qi and blood, resulting in chest pain. Phlegm turbidity moves with the upbearing and downbearing of the qi dynamic; it wants to exit the body, but cannot. This will cause panting and cough with rough breathing.

Thick, sticky yellow or white phlegm:
Evil heat scorches and damages the body fluids and causes them to be depleted. This results in thick, sticky phlegm. If the evil heat is deep within the body, the phlegm is yellow. If the evil heat is more superficial, the phlegm is white.

Somber facial complexion and dark purple lips:
Phlegm turbidity blocks the channels and network vessels, causing *qi* stagnation and blood stasis. If *qi* and blood are unable to nourish the head and face properly, the facial complexion will be somber, and the lips dark purple.

Pulse:
A slippery and rapid pulse.

Analysis

- The slippery pulse has a smooth onset and recession. It is smooth and evasive, like pearls rolling on a dish.
- The rapid pulse beats five or more times per respiration.

Liver Depression and *Qi* Stagnation

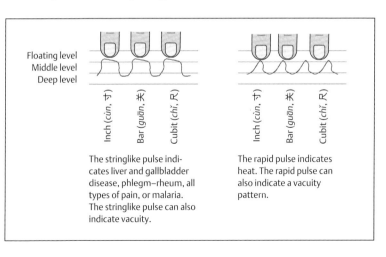

Floating level
Middle level
Deep level

Inch (*cùn*, 寸)   Bar (*guān*, 关)   Cubit (*chǐ*, 尺)

Inch (*cùn*, 寸)   Bar (*guān*, 关)   Cubit (*chǐ*, 尺)

The stringlike pulse indicates liver and gallbladder disease, phlegm–rheum, all types of pain, or malaria. The stringlike pulse can also indicate vacuity.

The rapid pulse indicates heat. The rapid pulse can also indicate a vacuity pattern.

Signs and symptoms

Bitter fullness in the chest and rib-side, vexation with rashness and irascibility, dizziness and tinnitus, a dry mouth, dry stools, short voidings of reddish urine, a red tongue with yellow tongue fur, and a rapid and stringlike pulse.

Bitter fullness in the chest and rib-side:
Liver depression and *qi* stagnation causes disharmony of the *qi* dynamic, resulting in gallbladder *qi* rising upward to invade the chest and diaphragm, which produces bitter fullness in the chest and rib-side.

Dizziness and tinnitus:
Heat evil congesting in the interior will travel along the channels and harass the upper body, clouding and blocking the clear orifices of the head and face. This will affect the normal upbearing and downbearing of the *qi* dynamic, and produce dizziness and tinnitus.

Vexation with rashness and irascibility:
Evil heat brewing internally harasses the heart spirit, producing vexation. If the liver's free coursing is disrupted, liver *qi* cannot flow smoothly; this leads to irascibility.

Short voidings of reddish urine:
Evil heat congesting in the interior wants to exit the body through the lower burner. This produces short voidings of reddish urine.

Dry mouth and dry stool:
Evil heat consumes and depletes the body fluids, causing dryness of the mouth. If the intestinal tract lacks the moisture of body fluids, there will be dry stool.

Pulse:
A rapid and stringlike pulse.

Analysis

- The stringlike pulse is long, and feels like the string of a musical instrument.
- The rapid pulse beats five or more times per respiration.

Cold–Rheum Obstructing the Lung

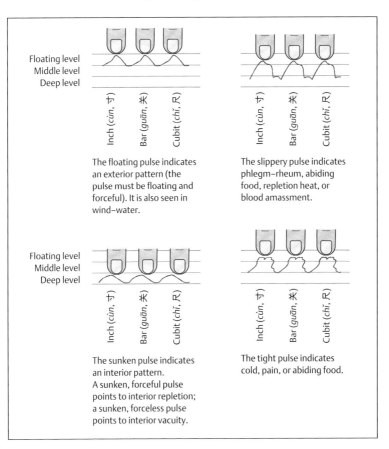

Floating level
Middle level
Deep level

Inch (*cùn*, 寸) Bar (*guān*, 关) Cubit (*chǐ*, 尺)

The floating pulse indicates an exterior pattern (the pulse must be floating and forceful). It is also seen in wind–water.

Inch (*cùn*, 寸) Bar (*guān*, 关) Cubit (*chǐ*, 尺)

The slippery pulse indicates phlegm–rheum, abiding food, repletion heat, or blood amassment.

Floating level
Middle level
Deep level

Inch (*cùn*, 寸) Bar (*guān*, 关) Cubit (*chǐ*, 尺)

The sunken pulse indicates an interior pattern.
A sunken, forceful pulse points to interior repletion; a sunken, forceless pulse points to interior vacuity.

Inch (*cùn*, 寸) Bar (*guān*, 关) Cubit (*chǐ*, 尺)

The tight pulse indicates cold, pain, or abiding food.

Signs and symptoms

Headache, severe cough and panting with an inability to lie flat that is mild during the day and worse at night, chest oppression, palpitations, copious thin white phlegm, a pale tongue with white or glossy slimy tongue fur, and a pulse that is floating and slippery, or sunken and tight.

Headache:

Water–rheum or cold evil congeals the *qi* and blood of the channels and network vessels, clouds and blocks the head, eyes, and clear orifices, and prevents the clear *yang qi* from ascending and descending. This produces headache.

Cough and panting:

Cold–rheum congesting in the lung impedes the normal upbearing and downbearing of the *qi* dynamic, thus producing cough. As phlegm-rheum moves with the upbearing and downbearing of the *qi* dynamic, it wants to exit the body but cannot; this causes panting.

Coughing and panting with an inability to lie flat that is mild during the day and worse at night:

Because there is an abundance of *yang qi* in the daytime, *yang qi* is able to pacify the *yin* cold evil, thereby resulting in milder symptoms during the day. Since there is more *yin qi* at night, the manifestations of *yin* cold are enhanced; therefore, the cough is more severe at night.

Chest oppression and palpitations:

Because of cold–rheum obstruction, the chest *yang* is devitalized, producing chest oppression. If cold–rheum invades the heart, the normal supply and distribution of heart blood will be disrupted, producing palpitations.

Copious thin white phlegm:

Cold rheum congeals, gathers, and floods upward into the mouth, producing copious, thin white phlegm.

Pulse:

A pulse that is floating and slippery, or sunken and tight.

Analysis

- The floating pulse is felt with light palpation. Although its strength is slightly reduced when heavy pressure is applied, it does not feel empty.
- The slippery pulse has a smooth onset and recession. It is smooth and evasive, like pearls rolling on a dish.
- The sunken pulse cannot be felt with light finger pressure. It is felt when heavy pressure is applied.
- The tight pulse is taut and tense. It feels like a pulled string or a twisted rope.

High Blood Pressure

Exuberant Internal Vacuity Cold, Counterflow Ascent of Phlegm Turbidity

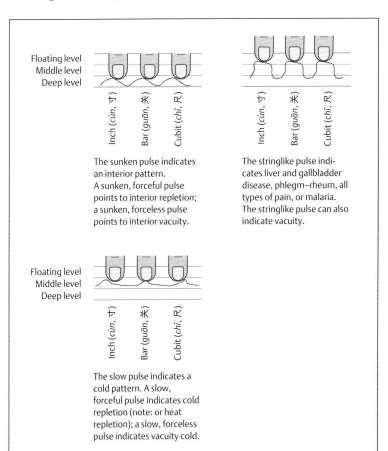

Floating level
Middle level
Deep level

Inch (*cùn*, 寸) Bar (*guān*, 关) Cubit (*chǐ*, 尺)

The sunken pulse indicates an interior pattern.
A sunken, forceful pulse points to interior repletion; a sunken, forceless pulse points to interior vacuity.

Inch (*cùn*, 寸) Bar (*guān*, 关) Cubit (*chǐ*, 尺)

The stringlike pulse indicates liver and gallbladder disease, phlegm–rheum, all types of pain, or malaria. The stringlike pulse can also indicate vacuity.

Floating level
Middle level
Deep level

Inch (*cùn*, 寸) Bar (*guān*, 关) Cubit (*chǐ*, 尺)

The slow pulse indicates a cold pattern. A slow, forceful pulse indicates cold repletion (note: or heat repletion); a slow, forceless pulse indicates vacuity cold.

Signs and symptoms

Headache (worse at the vertex), vexation and agitation, reversal cold of the extremities, dry retching or ejection of foamy drool, a pale enlarged tongue with tooth marks, white glossy slimy tongue fur, and a pulse that is sunken and stringlike, or sunken and slow.

Headache (worse at the vertex):
Both the bladder channel and the governing vessel transport *yang qi*. They also both meet at the vertex. Exuberant internal vacuity cold causes *yang qi* to be comparatively insufficient; thus, when there is a counterflow ascent of phlegm turbidity impeding the flow of *qi* and blood, there will be vertex headache that is especially severe.

Reversal cold of the extremities:
Debilitation of *yang qi* results in the lack of force needed to transport *qi* and blood to the four extremities. This leads to reversal cold of the extremities.

Vexation and agitation:
Phlegm turbidity harasses the heart spirit, causing vexation and agitation.

Dry retching or ejection of foamy drool:
Phlegm turbidity impairs the normal upbearing and downbearing of the *qi* dynamic, leading to a counterflow ascent of stomach *qi*. As a result, there is dry retching. If cold–rheum in the stomach follows the counterflow ascent of the *qi* dynamic, there will be ejection of foamy drool.

Pulse:
A pulse that is sunken and stringlike, or sunken and slow.

Analysis

- The sunken pulse cannot be felt with light finger pressure. It is felt when heavy pressure is applied.
- The stringlike pulse is long, and feels like the string of a musical instrument.
- The slow pulse has a slow onset and recession. It beats three times per respiration.

Liver Depression and Gallbladder Stagnation, Disharmony of the *Qi* Dynamic

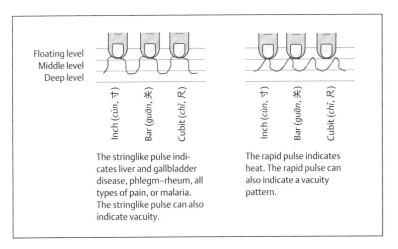

Floating level
Middle level
Deep level

Inch (*cùn*, 寸)   Bar (*guān*, 关)   Cubit (*chǐ*, 尺)

Inch (*cùn*, 寸)   Bar (*guān*, 关)   Cubit (*chǐ*, 尺)

The stringlike pulse indicates liver and gallbladder disease, phlegm–rheum, all types of pain, or malaria. The stringlike pulse can also indicate vacuity.

The rapid pulse indicates heat. The rapid pulse can also indicate a vacuity pattern.

Signs and symptoms

Bitter fullness in the chest and rib-side, vexation with rashness and irascibility, dizziness and tinnitus, dry mouth, dry stool, short voidings of reddish urine, a red tongue with yellow tongue fur, and a rapid and stringlike pulse.

Bitter fullness in the chest and rib-side:
Liver depression and gallbladder stagnation causes disharmony of the *qi* dynamic, resulting in gallbladder *qi* rising upward to invade the chest and diaphragm, which produces bitter fullness in the chest and rib-side.

Dizziness and tinnitus:
Heat evil congesting in the interior will travel along the channels and harass the upper body, clouding and blocking the clear orifices of the head and face. This will affect the normal upbearing and downbearing of the *qi* dynamic and produce dizziness and tinnitus.

Vexation with rashness and irascibility:
Evil heat consumes and depletes the body fluids, causing dryness of the mouth. If the intestinal tract lacks the moisture of body fluids, there will be dry stool.

Short voidings of reddish urine:
Evil heat congesting in the interior wants to exit the body through the lower bur-

ner. This produces short voidings of reddish urine.

Dry mouth and dry stool:
Evil heat brewing internally harasses the heart spirit, producing vexation. If the liver's free coursing is disrupted, liver *qi* cannot flow smoothly; this leads to irascibility.

Pulse;
A rapid and stringlike pulse.

Analysis

- The stringlike pulse is long, and feels like the string of a musical instrument.
- The rapid pulse beats five or more times per respiration.

■ Heart Disease

Water *Qi* Intimidating the Heart (Vacuity–Repletion Complex)

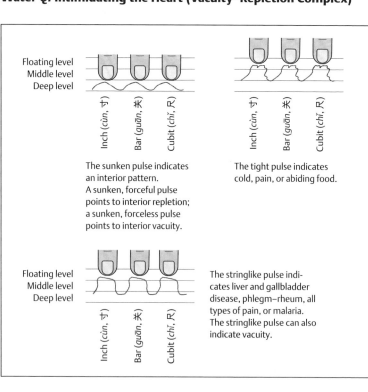

Floating level
Middle level
Deep level

Inch (cùn, 寸) Bar (guān, 关) Cubit (chǐ, 尺)

Inch (cùn, 寸) Bar (guān, 关) Cubit (chǐ, 尺)

The sunken pulse indicates an interior pattern.
A sunken, forceful pulse points to interior repletion; a sunken, forceless pulse points to interior vacuity.

The tight pulse indicates cold, pain, or abiding food.

Floating level
Middle level
Deep level

Inch (cùn, 寸) Bar (guān, 关) Cubit (chǐ, 尺)

The stringlike pulse indicates liver and gallbladder disease, phlegm–rheum, all types of pain, or malaria. The stringlike pulse can also indicate vacuity.

Signs and symptoms

Oppression and dull pain in the chest or severe pain in the chest and back, palpitations, dizzy vision, a pale enlarged tongue body with pronounced tooth marks, white moist tongue fur, and a pulse that is sunken and tight, or stringlike.

Oppression and dull pain in the chest or severe pain in the chest and back:
The counterflow ascent of water *qi* to the chest and diaphragm causes *qi* and blood stasis obstruction of the heart vessels.

Dizzy vision:
Water–rheum or dampness evil clouds and blocks the head, eyes, and clear orifices, and prevents the clear *yang qi* from ascending and descending. This results in dizzy vision.

Palpitations:
Water–rheum or dampness evil invading the heart obstructs the normal supply and distribution of heart blood, producing palpitations.

Pulse:
A pulse that is sunken and tight, or stringlike.

Analysis

- The sunken pulse cannot be felt with light finger pressure. It is felt when heavy pressure is applied.
- The stringlike pulse is long, and feels like the string of a musical instrument.
- The tight pulse is taut and tense. It feels like a pulled string or a twisted rope.

Debilitation of Kidney *Yang*, Cold Water Flooding Upward

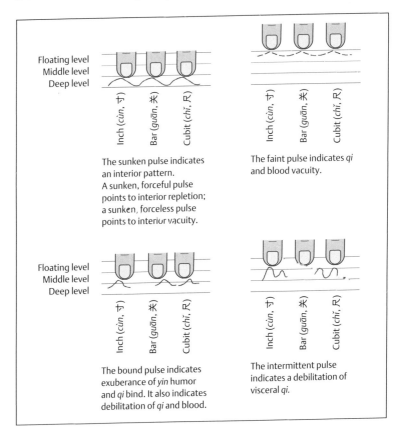

The sunken pulse indicates an interior pattern.
A sunken, forceful pulse points to interior repletion; a sunken, forceless pulse points to interior vacuity.

The faint pulse indicates *qi* and blood vacuity.

The bound pulse indicates exuberance of *yin* humor and *qi* bind. It also indicates debilitation of *qi* and blood.

The intermittent pulse indicates a debilitation of visceral *qi*.

Signs and symptoms

Dizziness, palpitations, chest pain stretching through to the back, physical cold and cold limbs, a pale moist tongue with white glossy tongue fur, and a pulse that is sunken and faint, or bound and intermittent.

Dizziness:
Water–rheum or dampness evil clouds and blocks the head, eyes, and clear orifices, and prevents the clear *yang qi* from ascending and descending. This results in dizziness.

Palpitations:
Water–rheum or dampness evil invades the heart, obstructing the normal supply and distribution of heart blood. This causes palpitations.

Chest pain stretching through to the back:
Kidney *yang* debilitation leads to exuberant internal *yin* cold binding and gathering in the chest and diaphragm. Channel *qi* and blood become congealed and stagnated as a result; when there is obstruction of *qi* and blood, there is pain.

Physical cold and cold limbs:
Debilitation of original *qi* leads to an insufficiency of *yang qi* to transport the *qi* and blood to the four limbs.

Pulse:
A pulse that is sunken and faint, or bound and intermittent.

Analysis

- The sunken pulse cannot be felt with light finger pressure. It is felt when heavy pressure is applied.
- The faint pulse is extremely thin and extremely soft. It is vague and indistinct, and has an unclear rate.
- The bound pulse is slow and sluggish, and pauses periodically at irregular intervals.
- The intermittent pulse pauses periodically at regular intervals.

Phlegm and Heat Binding Together, Obstruction of Heart *Yang*

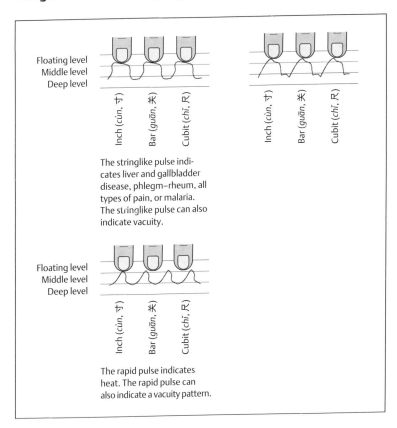

Floating level
Middle level
Deep level

Inch (cùn, 寸)   Bar (guān, 关)   Cubit (chǐ, 尺)

Inch (cùn, 寸)   Bar (guān, 关)   Cubit (chǐ, 尺)

The stringlike pulse indicates liver and gallbladder disease, phlegm–rheum, all types of pain, or malaria. The stringlike pulse can also indicate vacuity.

Floating level
Middle level
Deep level

Inch (cùn, 寸)   Bar (guān, 关)   Cubit (chǐ, 尺)

The rapid pulse indicates heat. The rapid pulse can also indicate a vacuity pattern.

Signs and symptoms

Glomus and fullness of the chest and stomach duct, phlegm rale, palpitations, constipation, a red-tipped tongue, yellow and slimy tongue fur, and a pulse that is slippery and stringlike, or rapid and stringlike.

Glomus and fullness of the chest and stomach duct:
Phlegm turbidity congesting in the chest and stomach duct blocks the normal upbearing and downbearing of stomach *yang*. As a result, there is glomus and fullness of the chest and stomach duct.

Phlegm rale and palpitations:
Phlegm–heat congests and blocks the heart and lungs. When the flow of heart *yang* is affected, there will be palpitations. If phlegm turbidity follows the upbearing or downbearing of the *qi* dynamic, there will be phlegm rale.

Constipation:
Phlegm–heat congests and blocks stomach *yang*, impairing the upbearing and downbearing of the *qi* dynamic of the intestinal tract. This impairs conveyance in the intestinal tract, resulting in constipation.

Pulse:
A pulse that is slippery and stringlike, or rapid and stringlike.
The slippery pulse indicates phlegm–rheum, abiding food, repletion heat, or blood amassment.

Analysis

- The stringlike pulse is long, and feels like the string of a musical instrument.
- The slippery pulse has a smooth onset and recession. It is smooth and evasive, like pearls rolling on a dish.
- The rapid pulse beats five or more times per respiration.

Insufficiency of *Qi* and Blood, Dual Vacuity of *Yin* and *Yang*

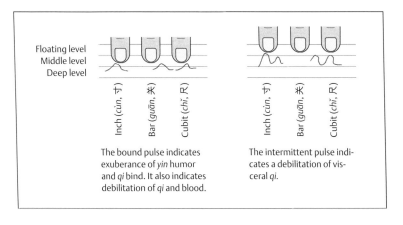

The bound pulse indicates exuberance of *yin* humor and *qi* bind. It also indicates debilitation of *qi* and blood.

The intermittent pulse indicates a debilitation of visceral *qi*.

Signs and symptoms

Chest oppression and pain, palpitations, shortage of *qi* and lack of strength, a pale tongue with moist white tongue fur, and a bound and intermittent pulse.

Chest oppression and pain:
When *yin*, *yang*, *qi*, and blood are insufficient, the heart and lung lack the force to move *qi* and blood. This results in the abnormal upbearing and downbearing of the *qi* dynamic, which congests and stagnates in the chest, causing chest oppression and pain.

Palpitations:
Insufficiency of *qi* and blood leads to debilitation of heart *yang*, which results in the inability to moisten and nourish the heart viscera. This causes palpitations.

Shortage of *qi* and lack of strength:
Insufficient production of *qi* and blood leads to *qi* weakness and blood vacuity. This causes shortage of *qi* and lack of strength.

Pulse:
A bound and intermittent pulse.

Analysis

- The bound pulse is slow and sluggish, and pauses periodically at irregular intervals.
- The intermittent pulse pauses periodically at regular intervals.

Gastric Ulcer

Liver and Stomach *Yin* Vacuity

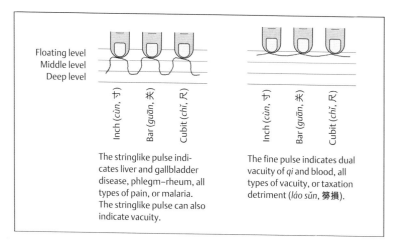

Floating level
Middle level
Deep level

Inch (*cùn*, 寸)   Bar (*guān*, 关)   Cubit (*chǐ*, 尺)

Inch (*cùn*, 寸)   Bar (*guān*, 关)   Cubit (*chǐ*, 尺)

The stringlike pulse indicates liver and gallbladder disease, phlegm–rheum, all types of pain, or malaria. The stringlike pulse can also indicate vacuity.

The fine pulse indicates dual vacuity of *qi* and blood, all types of vacuity, or taxation detriment (*láo sǔn*, 劳损).

Signs and symptoms

Dry mouth and throat, distending pain in the stomach duct, hypertonicity and pain in all four limbs, dry bound stools, a red and tender tongue tip that is lacking in moisture, and a fine, stringlike pulse.

Dry mouth and throat:
Depletion if internal *yin* humor causes an insufficiency of body fluids to moisten the throat and mouth, thus producing a dry mouth and throat.

Distending pain in the stomach duct:
An insufficient production of stomach fluids leads to a lack of moistening and nourishment of the *qi*, blood, channels, and network vessels. As a result, *qi* and blood will congeal and stagnate, causing distending pain of the stomach duct.

Hypertonicity and pain in the four limbs:
Qi stagnation and blood stasis result in insufficient *qi* and blood to moisten and nourish the sinews and vessels; thus, there is hypertonicity and pain of the four limbs.

Dry bound stool:
The depletion of *yin* humor in the intestinal tract causes a dry bound stool.

Pulse:
A fine and stringlike pulse.

Analysis

- The stringlike pulse is long, and feels like the string of a musical instrument.
- The fine pulse is thin (like a thread) yet clear.

Spleen–Stomach Vacuity Cold

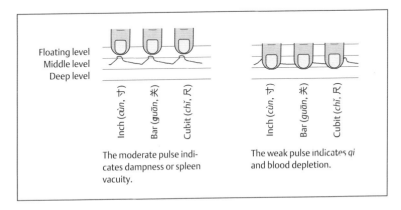

Floating level
Middle level
Deep level

Inch (cùn, 寸)   Bar (guān, 关)   Cubit (chǐ, 尺)

Inch (cùn, 寸)   Bar (guān, 关)   Cubit (chǐ, 尺)

The moderate pulse indicates dampness or spleen vacuity.

The weak pulse indicates qi and blood depletion.

Signs and symptoms

Glomus, fullness, and distending pain of the chest and stomach duct that likes pressure and warmth; an upwelling and vomiting of clear water; a bland taste in the mouth with torpid intake; lack of warmth in the extremities; sloppy, rotten stools; a pale, enlarged, tooth-marked tongue with white, moist, and slightly slimy tongue fur; and a moderate, weak pulse.

Glomus, fullness, and distending pain of the chest and stomach duct that likes pressure and warmth:
Spleen–stomach vacuity cold leads to *yin* cold evil congealing and gathering in the stomach duct and abdomen, which causes the flow of *qi* and blood to be congealed and stagnated as well. As a result, there is distending pain of the stomach duct. In addition, since the pathogen belongs to cold and vacuity, there is a preference for pressure and warmth.

Bland taste in the mouth and torpid intake:
Cold *qi* congealing and stagnating in the interior causes debilitation *of yang qi*. When *yang qi* is vacuous, it is unable to move and transform water-damp, resulting in a bland taste in the mouth. In

addition, spleen–stomach vacuity cold coupled with water–damp collecting in the stomach leads to torpid intake.

Upwelling and vomiting of clear water:
Spleen–stomach vacuity cold impairs the spleen's function of transformation and movement, and thus leads to water–rheum collecting in the stomach. When water–rheum follows the counter-flow ascent of stomach *qi*, there is an upwelling and vomiting of clear water.

Lack of warmth in the extremities:
Insufficiency of *yang qi* causes impaired flow of *qi* and blood in the channels and network vessels. *Qi* and blood are there-fore unable to reach the extremities.

Sloppy rotten stool:
Exuberant internal vacuity cold evil in-jures *yang qi*, causing a disturbance in the conveyance of the stomach and in-testines. As a result, there is a sloppy, rotten stool.

Pulse:
A moderate and weak pulse.

Analysis

- The moderate pulse is slightly faster than the slow pulse. It beats four times per respiration, and its arrival is leisurely.
- The weak pulse is sunken, soft, and thin.

Cold–Heat Complex (Vacuity-Repletion Complex)

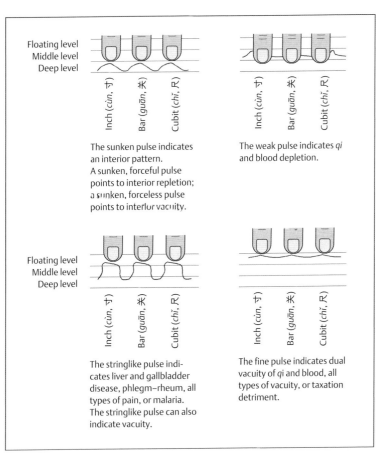

Floating level
Middle level
Deep level

Inch (cùn, 寸)
Bar (guān, 关)
Cubit (chǐ, 尺)

The sunken pulse indicates an interior pattern.
A sunken, forceful pulse points to interior repletion; a sunken, forceless pulse points to interior vacuity.

Inch (cùn, 寸)
Bar (guān, 关)
Cubit (chǐ, 尺)

The weak pulse indicates *qi* and blood depletion.

Floating level
Middle level
Deep level

Inch (cùn, 寸)
Bar (guān, 关)
Cubit (chǐ, 尺)

The stringlike pulse indicates liver and gallbladder disease, phlegm–rheum, all types of pain, or malaria. The stringlike pulse can also indicate vacuity.

Inch (cùn, 寸)
Bar (guān, 关)
Cubit (chǐ, 尺)

The fine pulse indicates dual vacuity of *qi* and blood, all types of vacuity, or taxation detriment.

Signs and symptoms

Vomiting, glomus and fullness or distending pain in the stomach duct, clamoring stomach, upflow of acid, hunger with no desire to eat, rumbling intestines and diarrhea, a pale and enlarged tongue with slimy, yellow (or white) tongue fur, and a pulse that is (a) sunken, (b) fine and weak, or (c) fine and stringlike.

Vomiting:
A mix of cold and heat in the stomach leads to impairment of the harmonious downbearing of the stomach. This, in turn, causes a counterflow ascent of stomach *qi*, and thus vomiting.

Glomus and fullness or distending pain in the stomach duct:
Binding cold and heat glomus in the stomach causes a disturbance in the spleen and stomach's ability to upbear the clear and downbear the turbid. As a result, there is glomus and fullness or distending pain in the stomach duct.

Clamoring stomach with acid upflow and hunger with no desire to eat:
A combination of cold and heat evil *qi* in the stomach leads to spleen–stomach disharmony; when liver *qi* invades the stomach, there is a clamoring stomach with acid upflow. If cold and heat evil obstructs the *qi* dynamic, the result is glomus and fullness of the stomach duct, which produces hunger with no desire to eat.

Rumbling intestines and diarrhea:
A disturbance in the upbearing and downbearing of the spleen–stomach's *qi* dynamic causes rumbling intestines. Water–damp pouring downward into the intestinal tract causes diarrhea.

Pulse:
A pulse that is (a) sunken, (b) fine and weak, or (c) fine and stringlike.

Analysis

- The sunken pulse cannot be felt with light finger pressure. It is felt when heavy pressure is applied.
- The weak pulse is sunken, soft, and thin.
- The stringlike pulse is long, and feels like the string of a musical instrument.
- The fine pulse is thin (like a thread) yet clear.

■ Liver Cirrhosis

Liver Depression and Damp Obstruction (Vacuity–Repletion Complex)

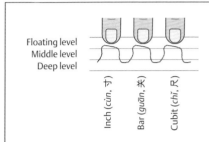

Floating level
Middle level
Deep level

Inch (cùn, 寸)
Bar (guān, 关)
Cubit (chǐ, 尺)

The stringlike pulse indicates liver and gallbladder disease, phlegm–rheum, all types of pain, or malaria. The stringlike pulse can also indicate vacuity.

Signs and symptoms

Dizzy head and vision, vexation with rashness and irascibility, rib-side pain, glomus and fullness of the chest and diaphragm, reduced food intake, distention after meals, short voidings of reddish urine, white glossy tongue fur, and a stringlike pulse.

Dizzy head and vision:
Constrained liver *qi* and an inhibited *qi* dynamic can lead to a failure of clear *yang* to ascend and turbid *qi* to descend, thus resulting in a dizzy head and vision.

Vexation with rashness and irascibility:
A long-term binding constraint of liver *qi* can transform into fire. If the internal stirring of vacuity fire rises upward to harass the heart spirit, there will be vexation with rashness and irascibility.

Rib-side pain:
The liver channel passes through the costal region; if there is stasis and ob-

struction of liver *qi*, there will be rib-side pain.

Short voidings of reddish urine:
Long-term congestion of the *qi* dynamic due to damp turbidity transforms into heat. Evil heat attempting to exit the body through the lower burner produces short voidings of reddish urine.

Reduced food intake and distention after meals:
Constrained liver *qi* and failure of the spleen to move and transform can lead to water–damp collecting in the middle burner, causing reduced food intake. Inhibited upbearing and downbearing of

the spleen and stomach's *qi* dynamic produces distention after meals.

Glomus and fullness of the chest and diaphragm:
Damp turbidity congestion in the chest and diaphragm leads to inhibited diffusion and downbearing of the *qi* dynamic, which produces glomus and fullness of the chest and diaphragm.

Pulse:
A stringlike pulse.

Analysis

- The stringlike pulse is long, and feels like the string of a musical instrument.

Damp-Heat Brewing Internally

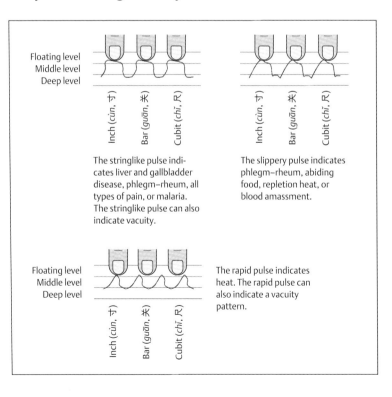

The stringlike pulse indicates liver and gallbladder disease, phlegm–rheum, all types of pain, or malaria. The stringlike pulse can also indicate vacuity.

The slippery pulse indicates phlegm–rheum, abiding food, repletion heat, or blood amassment.

The rapid pulse indicates heat. The rapid pulse can also indicate a vacuity pattern.

Signs and Symptoms

Nausea and vomiting, fever and thirst, yellowing of the body and eyes (resembling the color of a tangerine), distention and fullness in the abdomen, scanty yellow urine, constipation, a red tongue tip and margins, yellow slimy tongue fur, and a pulse that is rapid, slippery, and stringlike.

Nausea and vomiting:
Glomus and obstruction from damp–heat impairs the harmonious downbearing of the stomach. The resulting ascending counterflow of stomach *qi* causes nausea and vomiting.

Fever and thirst:
Intense heat evil in the body produces fever. If the damp–heat scorches and damages the body fluids, the resulting insufficiency of body fluids will produce thirst.

Yellowing of the body and eyes (resembling the color of a tangerine):
Damp–heat fumigating and steaming the interior combined with liver and gallbladder constraint transforming into heat results in the overflow and leakage of bile into the fleshy exterior. This produces yellowing of the body and eyes. In addition, since heat evil belongs to the category of *yang* evil, the color is bright yellow.

Distention and fullness in the abdomen:
Glomus and obstruction of damp–heat in the middle burner disturbs the upbearing and downbearing of the *qi* dynamic in the stomach and intestines. As a result, there is distention and fullness in the abdomen.

Constipation:
Due to damp–heat collecting in the interior, the upbearing and downbearing of the *qi* dynamic in the intestinal tract is disrupted. As a result, conveyance in the stomach and intestines is impaired.

Scanty yellow urine:
Damp–heat steams the interior, making it difficult for water–damp to be expelled. As a result, there is scanty urine. Since evil heat attempts to exit the body through the lower burner, the urine is yellow in color.

Pulse:
A pulse that is rapid, slippery, and stringlike.

Analysis

- The stringlike pulse is long, and feels like the string of a musical instrument.
- The slippery pulse has a smooth onset and recession. It is smooth and evasive, like pearls rolling on a dish.
- The rapid pulse beats five or more times per respiration.

Water–Rheum Collecting and Binding (Vacuity–Repletion Complex)

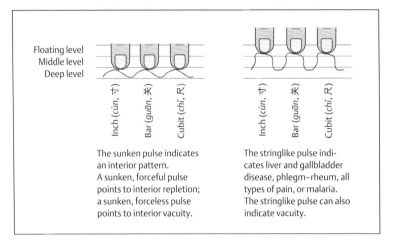

Floating level
Middle level
Deep level

Inch (cùn, 寸)   Bar (guān, 关)   Cubit (chǐ, 尺)

The sunken pulse indicates an interior pattern. A sunken, forceful pulse points to interior repletion; a sunken, forceless pulse points to interior vacuity.

Inch (cùn, 寸)   Bar (guān, 关)   Cubit (chǐ, 尺)

The stringlike pulse indicates liver and gallbladder disease, phlegm–rheum, all types of pain, or malaria. The stringlike pulse can also indicate vacuity.

Signs and symptoms

Oppression and pain in the chest and rib-side, an enlarged abdomen with glomus and fullness, abdominal distention that is worse after meals, nausea and vomiting, shortness of breath, short voidings of reddish urine, white glossy tongue fur, and a pulse that is sunken and stringlike.

Oppression and pain in the chest and rib-side:

The liver channel passes through the rib-side region; if the liver's free coursing is impaired due to water–rheum obstruction, *qi* and blood flow will be inhibited,

and there will be oppression and pain in the chest and rib-side.

Nausea and vomiting:

Glomus and obstruction from damp turbidity impairs the harmonious downbearing of the stomach. The resulting ascending counterflow of stomach *qi* causes nausea and vomiting .

Shortness of breath:
Water–rheum collecting in the body and invades the lung, causing failure of the lung to diffuse and downbear. As a result, there is shortness of breath.

An enlarged abdomen with glomus and fullness, and abdominal distention that is worse after meals:
Binding constraint of damp–heat in the middle burner causes distention and full-

ness in the abdominal region. If the diffusion and downbearing of the *qi* dynamic is inhibited, there will be abdominal distention that is worse after meals.

Short voidings of reddish urine:
Internal exuberant water–damp impairs the triple burner's function of keeping the sluices clear. As a result, damp–heat brews internally, causing short voidings of reddish urine.

Pulse:
A sunken and stringlike pulse.

Analysis

- The sunken pulse cannot be felt with light finger pressure. It is felt when heavy pressure is applied.
- The stringlike pulse is long, and feels like the string of a musical instrument.

■ Chronic Hepatitis

Liver Depression and *Qi* Stagnation

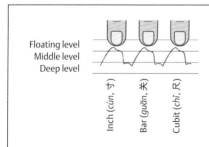

Floating level
Middle level
Deep level

Inch (cùn, 寸)
Bar (guān, 关)
Cubit (chǐ, 尺)

The stringlike pulse indicates liver and gallbladder disease, phlegm–rheum, all types of pain, or malaria. The stringlike pulse can also indicate vacuity.

Signs and symptoms

A bitter taste in the mouth, rib-side distention and pain, hepatomegaly, glomus of the stomach duct, abdominal distention, white and yellow tongue fur, and a stringlike pulse.

Bitter taste in the mouth:

Impairment of the liver's function of free coursing leads to liver *qi* depression and stagnation; gallbladder *qi* will flow up into the mouth, producing a bitter taste there.

Rib-side distention and pain with hepatomegaly:

The liver channel passes through the rib-side region. If the liver's free coursing is disturbed, *qi* and blood flow will be inhibited, resulting in liver depression and blood stasis. This causes rib-side distention and pain or hepatomegaly.

Glomus of the stomach duct and abdominal distention:

A disturbance in the liver's function of free coursing causes the *qi* dynamic of the spleen–stomach to congest in the stomach duct and the abdomen to be distended, resulting in distention and fullness in the abdominal region.

Pulse:

A stringlike pulse.

Analysis

- The stringlike pulse is long, and feels like the string of a musical instrument.

Cold–Damp Obstructing the Center (Vacuity-Repletion Complex)

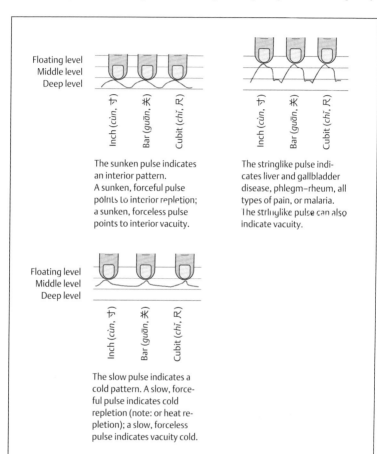

Floating level
Middle level
Deep level

Inch (cùn, 寸)   Bar (guān, 关)   Cubit (chǐ, 尺)

The sunken pulse indicates an interior pattern. A sunken, forceful pulse points to interior repletion; a sunken, forceless pulse points to interior vacuity.

Inch (cùn, 寸)   Bar (guān, 关)   Cubit (chǐ, 尺)

The stringlike pulse indicates liver and gallbladder disease, phlegm–rheum, all types of pain, or malaria. The stringlike pulse can also indicate vacuity.

Floating level
Middle level
Deep level

Inch (cùn, 寸)   Bar (guān, 关)   Cubit (chǐ, 尺)

The slow pulse indicates a cold pattern. A slow, forceful pulse indicates cold repletion (note: or heat repletion); a slow, forceless pulse indicates vacuity cold.

Signs and symptoms

Dark and gloomy yellowing of the body that resembles the color of smoke, reduced food intake with oppression in the stomach duct, fear of cold and cold limbs, sloppy diarrhea, yellow urine, a pale tongue with white glossy tongue fur, and a pulse that is sunken and stringlike, or sunken and slow.

Dark and gloomy yellowing of the body that resembles the color of smoke:

Cold–damp evil blocks the biliary tract and causes the bile to overflow and leak into the fleshy exterior, producing a dark and gloomy yellowing of the body. Since cold–damp evil is a *yin* evil, the yellow resembles the color of smoke.

Fear of cold and cold limbs:

Internal exuberant cold–damp causes a relative insufficiency of *yang qi*. This insufficiency leads to an inability of *qi* and blood to reach the four limbs, resulting in a fear of cold and cold limbs.

Sloppy diarrhea:

Cold–damp glomus and obstruction in the middle burner causes spleen–stomach vacuity cold. When the spleen fails to move and transform, damp turbidity pours downward into the intestinal tract, producing sloppy diarrhea.

Reduced food intake with oppression in the stomach duct:

Cold–damp glomus and obstruction in the middle burner causes congestion and stagnation of the spleen–stomach's *qi* dynamic, resulting in reduced food intake with oppression in the stomach duct.

Pulse:

A pulse that is sunken and stringlike, or sunken and slow.

Analysis

- The sunken pulse cannot be felt with light finger pressure. It is felt when heavy pressure is applied.
- The stringlike pulse is long, and feels like the string of a musical instrument.
- The slow pulse has a slow onset and recession. It beats three times per respiration.

■ Diabetes

Intense Stomach Heat

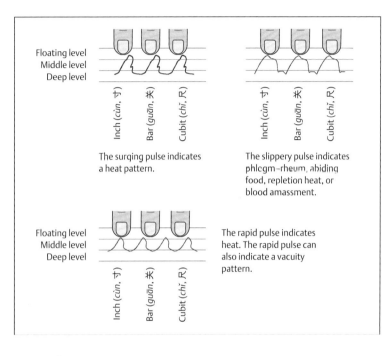

Floating level
Middle level
Deep level

Inch (cùn, 寸)   Bar (guān, 关)   Cubit (chǐ, 尺)

The surging pulse indicates a heat pattern.

Inch (cùn, 寸)   Bar (guān, 关)   Cubit (chǐ, 尺)

The slippery pulse indicates phlegm–rheum, abiding food, repletion heat, or blood amassment.

Floating level
Middle level
Deep level

Inch (cùn, 寸)   Bar (guān, 关)   Cubit (chǐ, 尺)

The rapid pulse indicates heat. The rapid pulse can also indicate a vacuity pattern.

Signs and symptoms

Great thirst with fluid intake, increased eating with rapid hungering, sweating, reddish urine, vexation, a red tongue with dry yellow tongue fur, and a pulse that is surging and large, or slippery and rapid.

Great thirst:
Intense stomach heat scorches and damages the body fluids. Insufficiency of the body fluids causes great thirst.

Sweating:
Intense interior heat forces body fluids to seep out of the body through the fleshy exterior; thus, there is sweating.

Vexation:
Heat evil rises upward to harass the heart spirit, causing vexation.

Increased eating with rapid hungering:
Intense evil heat in the stomach has a tendency to produce rapid digestion of the five grains, causing increased food intake with rapid hungering.

Short voidings of reddish urine:
Evil heat congests and obstructs the interior; it attempts to exit the body through the lower burner, thus producing short voidings of reddish urine.

Pulse:
A pulse that is surging and large, or slippery and rapid.

Analysis

- The surging pulse is huge; it has a strong onset and weak recession.
- The slippery pulse has a smooth onset and recession. It is smooth and evasive, like pearls rolling on a dish.
- The rapid pulse beats five or more times per respiration.

Yin Humor Depletion

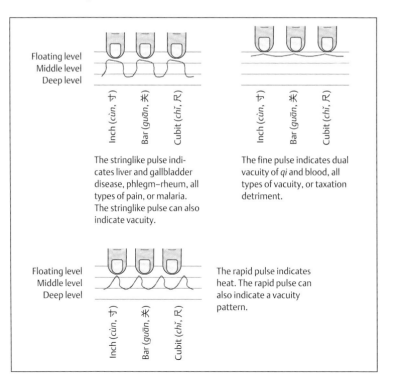

The stringlike pulse indicates liver and gallbladder disease, phlegm–rheum, all types of pain, or malaria. The stringlike pulse can also indicate vacuity.

The fine pulse indicates dual vacuity of *qi* and blood, all types of vacuity, or taxation detriment.

The rapid pulse indicates heat. The rapid pulse can also indicate a vacuity pattern.

Signs and symptoms

Thirst with increased fluid intake, dry throat, vexation and agitation, pain and hypertonicity of the limbs, dry stools, short voidings of scant urine, a dry red tongue with scant tongue fur, and a pulse that is stringlike and fine, or rapid, fine and forceless.

Thirst with increased fluid intake and dry throat:
Depletion of *yin* humor causes the body fluids to be insufficient and therefore unable to supply the throat and mouth. As a result, there is thirst with increased fluid intake and a dry throat.

Vexation and agitation:
Yin and blood vacuity in the body leads to the internal generation of vacuity heat. Vacuity heat harasses and stirs the heart spirit; when the heart is deprived of nourishment, there is vexation and agitation.

Pain and hypertonicity of the limbs:
A depletion of *yin* humor in the body leads to insufficient *qi* and blood to moisten and nourish the sinews, causing pain and hypertonicity of the limbs.

Dry stools:
Insufficient *yin* humor in the body leads to the internal generation of vacuity fire. Vacuity fire scorches and damages the body fluids, causing desiccation of the intestinal fluids. As a result, there are dry stools.

Short voidings of reddish urine:
Depletion of *yin* humor in the body deprives the urinary bladder of body fluids to transform, producing short voidings of reddish urine.

Pulse:
A pulse that is stringlike and fine, or rapid, fine and forceless.

Analysis

- The stringlike pulse is long, and feels like the string of a musical instrument.
- The fine pulse is thin (like a thread) yet clear.
- The rapid pulse beats five or more times per respiration.

Binding of Dampness and Heat (Vacuity–Repletion Complex)

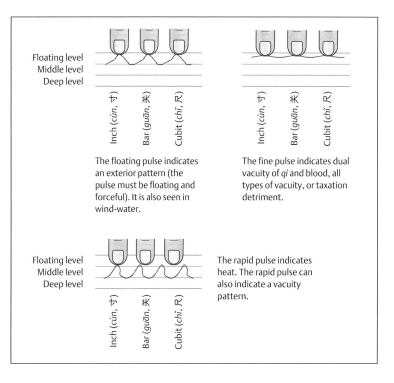

Floating level
Middle level
Deep level

Inch (*cùn*, 寸)   Bar (*guān*, 关)   Cubit (*chǐ*, 尺)

The floating pulse indicates an exterior pattern (the pulse must be floating and forceful). It is also seen in wind-water.

Inch (*cùn*, 寸)   Bar (*guān*, 关)   Cubit (*chǐ*, 尺)

The fine pulse indicates dual vacuity of *qi* and blood, all types of vacuity, or taxation detriment.

Floating level
Middle level
Deep level

Inch (*cùn*, 寸)   Bar (*guān*, 关)   Cubit (*chǐ*, 尺)

The rapid pulse indicates heat. The rapid pulse can also indicate a vacuity pattern.

Signs and symptoms

Thirst with increased fluid intake, increased eating with rapid hungering, vexation and insomnia, inhibited urination, diarrhea, a red tongue with scanty or no tongue fur, and a pulse that is floating and rapid, or fine and rapid.

Thirst with increased fluid intake:
Dampness and heat bind together, and the evil heat scorches and damages the body fluids, giving rise to thirst with increased fluid intake.

Increased eating with rapid hungering:
Evil heat congesting and stagnating in the stomach produces intense interior heat, which causes swift digestion and rapid hungering.

Vexation and insomnia:
Liver blood insufficiency leads to the internal generation of vacuity heat. Vacuity heat harasses and stirs the heart spirit, producing vexation. In addition, if there is lack of interaction between the heart

spirit and kidney *yin* due to kidney *yin* depletion, there will also be insomnia.

Inhibited urination:

Dampness and heat bind together and congest and block the lower burner, impairing the lower burner *qi* dynamic and the waterways. As a result, there is inhibited urination.

Diarrhea:

Damp–heat collects in the interior and pours downward into the large intestine, giving rise to diarrhea.

Pulse:

A pulse that is floating and rapid, or fine and rapid.

Analysis

- The floating pulse is felt with light palpation. Although its strength is slightly reduced when heavy pressure is applied, it does not feel empty.
- The fine pulse is thin (like a thread) yet clear.
- The rapid pulse beats five or more times per respiration.

Interior Heat Binding and Gathering

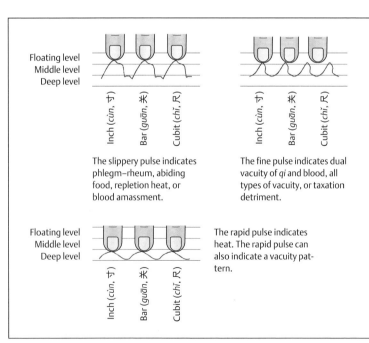

Floating level
Middle level
Deep level

Inch (*cùn*, 寸)   Bar (*guān*, 关)   Cubit (*chǐ*, 尺)

The slippery pulse indicates phlegm–rheum, abiding food, repletion heat, or blood amassment.

Inch (*cùn*, 寸)   Bar (*guān*, 关)   Cubit (*chǐ*, 尺)

The fine pulse indicates dual vacuity of *qi* and blood, all types of vacuity, or taxation detriment.

Floating level
Middle level
Deep level

Inch (*cùn*, 寸)   Bar (*guān*, 关)   Cubit (*chǐ*, 尺)

The rapid pulse indicates heat. The rapid pulse can also indicate a vacuity pattern.

Signs and symptoms

Vexation and thirst with increased intake of fluids, a dry mouth and tongue, increased eating with rapid hungering, tidal fever with sweating, fullness, distention, and pain of the abdomen, constipation, short voidings of reddish urine, a red tongue with dry yellow tongue fur or prickles, and a pulse that is slippery and rapid, or sunken, replete, and forceful.

Vexation and thirst with increased intake of fluids and a dry mouth and tongue:
Heat evil scorches and damages the body fluids. Depletion of the body fluids causes vexation and thirst with increased intake of fluids and dry mouth and tongue.

Tidal fever with sweating:
Intense interior heat forces the body fluids to exit through the fleshy exterior, leading to depletion of *yin* humor, which causes tidal fever with sweating.

Increased eating with rapid hungering:
Evil heat congesting and stagnating in the stomach produces intense interior heat, which causes swift digestion and rapid hungering.

Fullness, distention and pain of the abdomen:
Depletion of the body fluids causes dry bound stools in the intestinal tract. The normal upbearing and downbearing of the *qi* dynamic of the stomach and intestines are then disrupted, producing fullness, distention and pain of the abdomen.

Constipation and short voidings of reddish urine:
Evil heat scorches and damages the body fluids, which causes insufficiency of the fluids in the intestinal tract. This, in turn, causes the internal generation of vacuity heat. The scanty body fluids follow the evil heat into the urinary bladder, resulting in constipation and short voidings of reddish urine.

Pulse:
A pulse that is slippery and rapid, or sunken, replete, and forceful.

Analysis

- The slippery pulse has a smooth onset and recession. It is smooth and evasive, like pearls rolling on a dish.
- The fine pulse is thin (like a thread) yet clear.
- The rapid pulse beats five or more times per respiration.

Blood Stasis and Stomach Heat

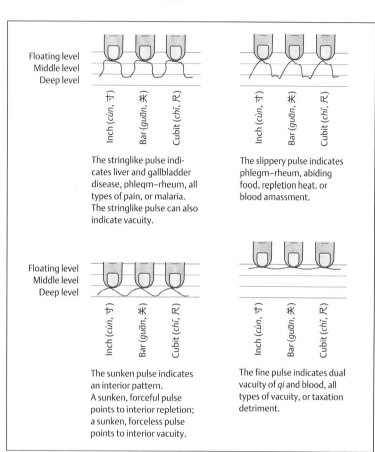

Floating level
Middle level
Deep level

Inch (*cùn*, 寸)   Bar (*guān*, 关)   Cubit (*chǐ*, 尺)

Inch (*cùn*, 寸)   Bar (*guān*, 关)   Cubit (*chǐ*, 尺)

The stringlike pulse indicates liver and gallbladder disease, phleqm–rheum, all types of pain, or malaria. The stringlike pulse can also indicate vacuity.

The slippery pulse indicates phlegm–rheum, abiding food, repletion heat. or blood amassment.

Floating level
Middle level
Deep level

Inch (*cùn*, 寸)   Bar (*guān*, 关)   Cubit (*chǐ*, 尺)

Inch (*cùn*, 寸)   Bar (*guān*, 关)   Cubit (*chǐ*, 尺)

The sunken pulse indicates an interior pattern. A sunken, forceful pulse points to interior repletion; a sunken, forceless pulse points to interior vacuity.

The fine pulse indicates dual vacuity of *qi* and blood, all types of vacuity, or taxation detriment.

Signs and symptoms

Thirst without increased intake of fluids, fatigue, paralysis of the four limbs, constipation with hard or bound stools, a dark purple tongue with thin yellow or white tongue fur, and a pulse that is stringlike and slippery, or sunken and fine.

Thirst without increased intake of fluids:

Evil heat scorching and damaging the body fluids produces thirst. A long-term brewing and accumulation of evil heat can injure construction blood.

Fatigue:

Dampness evil is heavy and turbid by nature; when it is combined with evil heat brewing and binding in the stomach and intestines, the spleen's function of movement and transformation is impaired. The resulting insufficient *qi* and blood formation causes fatigue.

Paralysis of the four limbs:

Evil heat and static blood bind together and inhibit the flow of *qi* and blood. As a result, the sinews are deprived of nourishment; thus, there is paralysis of the four limbs.

Constipation with hard or bound stools:

Evil heat brewing internally scorches and damages the *yin* humor, leading to insufficient body fluids; as a result, the stools are hard. If there is desiccation of the fluids of the intestinal tract, there will be constipation with bound stools.

Pulse:

A pulse that is stringlike and slippery, or sunken and fine.

Analysis

- The stringlike pulse is long, and feels like the string of a musical instrument.
- The slippery pulse has a smooth onset and recession. It is smooth and evasive, like pearls rolling on a dish.
- The sunken pulse cannot be felt with light finger pressure. It is felt when heavy pressure is applied.
- The fine pulse is thin (like a thread) yet clear.

■ Chronic Nephritis

Kidney Vacuity with Damp Depression, and Binding of Water and Heat (Vacuity–Repletion Complex)

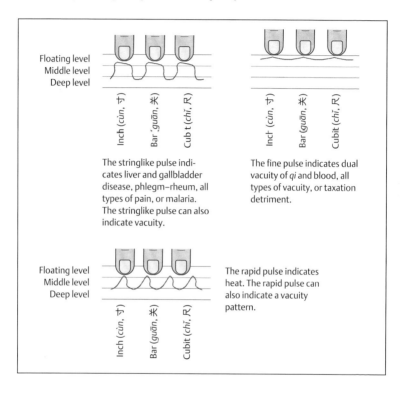

Floating level
Middle level
Deep level

Inch (cùn, 寸)
Bar (guān, 关)
Cubit (chǐ, 尺)

The stringlike pulse indicates liver and gallbladder disease, phlegm–rheum, all types of pain, or malaria. The stringlike pulse can also indicate vacuity.

Inch (cùn, 寸)
Bar (guān, 关)
Cubit (chǐ, 尺)

The fine pulse indicates dual vacuity of *qi* and blood, all types of vacuity, or taxation detriment.

Floating level
Middle level
Deep level

Inch (cùn, 寸)
Bar (guān, 关)
Cubit (chǐ, 尺)

The rapid pulse indicates heat. The rapid pulse can also indicate a vacuity pattern.

Signs and symptoms

Dizziness and tinnitus, a limp aching lumbus and knees, a puffy face and swelling of the feet, frequent but incomplete urination that is worse at night, low-grade fever, vexing heat in the five centers, a red tongue with scant tongue fur or a pale tongue with white tongue fur, and a pulse that is stringlike, fine, and rapid.

Limp aching lumbus and knees:
The lumbus is the house of the kidney; insufficiency of original *qi* due to kidney vacuity causes *qi*, blood, and sinews to be deprived of moisture and nourishment. As a result, there is a limp, aching lumbus and knees.

Vexing heat in the five centers:
Depletion of kidney *yin* causes vacuity fire to flame upward and damage the *yin* humor. As a result, there is vexing heat in the five centers.

Frequent but incomplete urination:
Damp–heat congesting and binding in the lower burner impairs bladder *qi* transformation, leading to inhibition of the waterways. As a result, there is frequent but incomplete urination.

Dizziness and tinnitus:
Insufficiency of kidney essence is unable to fill and nourish the sea of marrow (*suǐ hǎi*, 髓海), giving rise to dizziness and tinnitus.

Low-grade fever:
Damp–heat blocks the normal diffusion and downbearing of the *qi* dynamic. Damp–heat evil congeals and gathers in the body, producing a continuous low-grade fever that is difficult to eradicate.

Puffy face and swelling of the feet:
Kidney *yang* debilitation leads to disturbance of bladder *qi* transformation, which causes damp turbidity to collect and stagnate in the interior. Water–rheum overflowing and seeping into the head, face, and four limbs causes facial puffiness and swelling of the feet.

Pulse:
A pulse that is stringlike, fine, and rapid.

Analysis

- The stringlike pulse is long, and feels like the string of a musical instrument.
- The fine pulse is thin (like a thread) yet clear.
- The rapid pulse beats five or more times per respiration.

Lower Burner Damp–Heat and Water Amassment in the Bladder

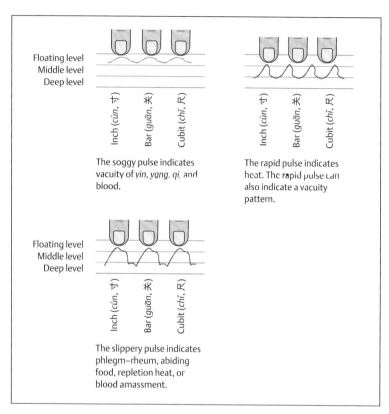

Floating level
Middle level
Deep level

Inch (cùn, 寸)   Bar (guān, 关)   Cubit (chǐ, 尺)

The soggy pulse indicates vacuity of yin, yang, qi, and blood.

Floating level
Middle level
Deep level

Inch (cùn, 寸)   Bar (guān, 关)   Cubit (chǐ, 尺)

The rapid pulse indicates heat. The rapid pulse can also indicate a vacuity pattern.

Floating level
Middle level
Deep level

Inch (cùn, 寸)   Bar (guān, 关)   Cubit (chǐ, 尺)

The slippery pulse indicates phlegm–rheum, abiding food, repletion heat, or blood amassment.

Signs and symptoms

Thirst, fever, fear of cold, urinary frequency, urinary urgency, painful or incessant dribbling urination, distending pain in the lesser abdomen, aching pain in the lumbus, thin yellow tongue fur, and a pulse that is soggy and rapid, or slippery and rapid.

Thirst:
Interior congestion and obstruction of damp–heat leads to difficulty in distributing the body fluids to the upper body. As a result, there is thirst.

Fever and fear of cold:
Damp–heat brewing internally and long-term depression will transform into fire. When fire heat evil steams and fumigates the interior, there is fever. Also, since fire–heat has a tendency to consume *qi* and *yin*, there will, if fire–heat evil injures the defense *qi*, be insufficient defense *qi* to warm the fleshy exterior, resulting in a fear of cold.

Urinary frequency, urinary urgency, painful or incessant dribbling urination:
Damp–heat binding and gathering in the lower burner impairs the bladder's *qi* transformation and disturbs the waterways. As a result, there is urinary frequency, urinary urgency, painful urination, and incessant dribbling urination.

Distending pain in the lesser abdomen and aching pain in the lumbus:
Damp–heat congestion and obstruction in the stomach duct and abdomen impairs the spleen–stomach's ability to upbear the clear and downbear the turbid. As a result, there is distending pain in the lesser abdomen.

Pulse:
A pulse that is soggy and rapid, or slippery and rapid.

Analysis

- The soggy pulse is floating, thin and soft.
- The rapid pulse beats five or more times per respiration.
- The slippery pulse has a smooth onset and recession. It is smooth and evasive, like pearls rolling on a dish.

■ Sciatica

Enduring Impediment Entering the Network Vessels

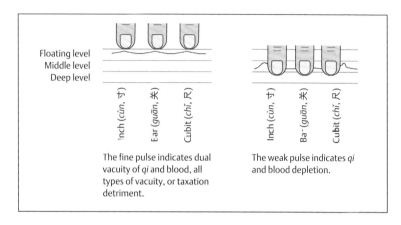

Floating level
Middle level
Deep level

Inch (cùn, 寸) Ear (guān, 关) Cubit (chǐ, 尺)

The fine pulse indicates dual vacuity of *qi* and blood, all types of vacuity, or taxation detriment.

Inch (cùn, 寸) Ba⁻ (guān, 关) Cubit (chǐ, 尺)

The weak pulse indicates *qi* and blood depletion.

Signs and symptoms

Prolonged pain in the lumbus and legs, gradual emaciation of the flesh with numbness and inhibited bending and stretching, difficult mobility, cold and fatigued limbs, a pale tongue with thin white tongue fur, and a fine, weak pulse.

Pain in the lumbus and legs:
Qi and blood vacuity deprives the sinews and bones of moisture and nourishment, which leads to wind–cold–damp evil stagnating in the sinews and bones. This produces lingering pain in the lumbus and legs.

Gradual emaciation of the flesh with numbness:
The spleen governs the flesh. If wind–cold–damp evil collects in the body and forms an impediment pattern (*bì zhèng*, 痹證), blocking the spleen's function

of movement and transformation, *qi* and blood will over time become even more vacuous. This will result in gradual emaciation of the flesh with numbness.

Inhibited bending and stretching with difficult mobility:
Wind–cold–damp evil blocks the flow of *qi* and blood in the channels and network vessels, causing the limbs and the blood vessels to be deprived of moisture and nourishment. This results in inhibited bending and stretching with difficult mobility.

Cold and fatigued limbs:
Wind–damp–cold evil congeals and stagnates in the flesh, inhibiting the movement of *qi* and blood. *Qi* and blood can no longer warm and nourish the four limbs, resulting in cold and fatigued limbs.

Pulse:
A fine, weak pulse.

Analysis

- The fine pulse is thin (like a thread) yet clear.
- The weak pulse is felt at the deep level. It is soft and forceless.

Water–Damp Invasion

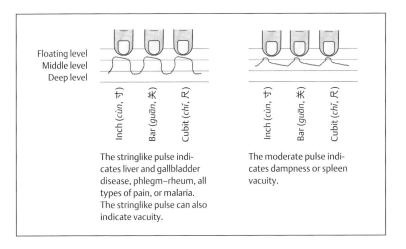

Floating level
Middle level
Deep level

Inch (*cùn*, 寸) Bar (*guān*, 夫) Cubit (*chǐ*, 尺)

Inch (*cùn*, 寸) Bar (*guān*, 夫) Cubit (*chǐ*, 尺)

The stringlike pulse indicates liver and gallbladder disease, phlegm–rheum, all types of pain, or malaria. The stringlike pulse can also indicate vacuity.

The moderate pulse indicates dampness or spleen vacuity.

Signs and symptoms

Stiffness and pain in the lumbus and legs with inhibited bending and stretching, pain upon exposure to cold that is relieved by heat, thin white tongue fur, and a moderate, stringlike pulse.

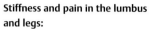

Stiffness and pain in the lumbus and legs:
Cold evil is a *yin* evil, and is, therefore, congealing and stagnating by nature. Cold evil blocks the movement of *qi* and blood in the channels and network vessels, and thus produces stiffness and pain in the lumbus and legs.

Inhibited bending and stretching:
Cold evil blocks the movement of *qi* and blood in the channels and network vessels. As a result, *qi* and blood can no longer warm and nourish the limbs, leading to inhibited bending and stretching of the lumbus and legs.

Pain upon exposure to cold that is relieved by heat:
When cold evil is exposed to heat, it will naturally be warmed and scattered. The circulation of *qi* and blood is normalized, and the pain is temporarily relieved. However, exposure to cold will cause *qi* and blood circulation to congeal and stagnate, resulting in exacerbation of the pain.

Pulse:
A moderate, stringlike pulse.

Analysis

- The stringlike pulse is long, and feels like the string of a musical instrument.
- The moderate pulse is slightly faster than the slow pulse. It beats four times per respiration, and its arrival is leisurely.

Congealing Phlegm–Damp

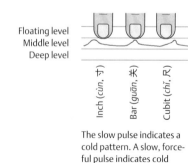

The slow pulse indicates a cold pattern. A slow, forceful pulse indicates cold repletion (note: or repletion heat); a slow, forceless pulse indicates vacuity cold.

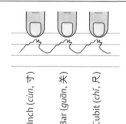

The rough pulse indicates damaged essence, blood vacuity, *qi* stagnation, or blood stasis.

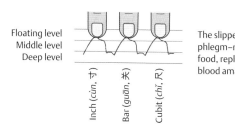

Floating level
Middle level
Deep level

Inch (cùn, 寸)   Bar (guān, 关)   Cubit (chǐ, 尺)

The slippery pulse indicates phlegm–rheum, abiding food, repletion heat, or blood amassment.

Signs and symptoms

Lumbar pain of fixed location that is worse at night, numbness, a heavy and cumbersome lumbus and legs, thick slimy tongue fur, and a pulse that is slow and rough, or slippery.

Lumbar pain of fixed location that is worse at night:

When phlegm and dampness congeal and bind together, *qi* and blood circulation stagnates. When there is obstruction of *qi* and blood, there is pain. Since dampness evil by nature is heavy and turbid, the lumbar pain is of fixed location. Dampness evil is a *yin* evil; as the night approaches, there is an increase in *yin* cold *qi*, which accounts for the worsening of the pain at night.

Numbness:

When phlegm and dampness congeal and bind together, *qi* and blood flow is inhibited. As a result, the sinews are deprived of moisture and nourishment, producing numbness of the four limbs.

Heavy and cumbersome lumbus and legs:

Dampness evil is heavy and turbid by nature. When *qi* and blood of the channels and network vessels are obstructed and stagnated by dampness evil, *qi* and blood circulation becomes inhibited. This causes a heavy and cumbersome lumbus and legs.

Pulse:

A pulse that is slow and rough, or slippery.

Analysis

- The slow pulse has a slow onset and recession. It beats three times per respiration.

- The rough pulse is slow, thin, and short. It has a harsh onset and recession.
- The slippery pulse has a smooth onset and recession. It is smooth and evasive, like pearls rolling on a dish.

■ Dysmenorrhea

Liver Depression and *Qi* Stagnation

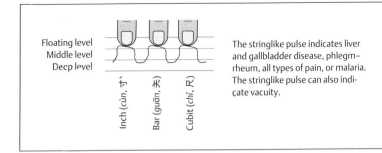

Floating level
Middle level
Deep level

Inch (*cùn*, 寸)

Bar (*guān*, 关)

Cubit (*chǐ*, 尺)

The stringlike pulse indicates liver and gallbladder disease, phlegm–rheum, all types of pain, or malaria. The stringlike pulse can also indicate vacuity.

Signs and symptoms

Distending pain in the lower abdomen before or during menstruation, scant menstrual flow or inhibited menstruation; distention and oppression in the chest and rib-side, frequent sighing, premenstrual vexation, agitation, and irascibility, breast distention, a dull and stagnant-looking tongue with white tongue fur, and a stringlike pulse.

Distending pain in the lower abdomen, scant menstrual flow, or inhibited menstruation:

The liver channel passes through the lesser abdominal region. Stasis obstruction of liver *qi* impairs the spleen–stomach's function of upbearing the clear and downbearing the turbid, resulting in distending pain in the lower abdomen, scant menstrual flow, or inhibited menstruation.

Distention and oppression in the chest and rib-side:

The liver channel passes through the chest and rib-side regions. Stasis obstruction of liver *qi* impairs the liver's function of free coursing, thus resulting in rib-side distention and oppression.

Frequent sighing:

Stasis obstruction of liver *qi* leads to inhibited upbearing and downbearing of the *qi* dynamic. Sighing relieves the congestion and stagnation of the *qi* dynamic, hence those with liver depression will present with frequent sighing.

Premenstrual vexation, agitation, and irascibility:

During the premenstrual period, a woman's *qi* and blood are preparing to rid of the old and engender the new. If her constitution is that of blood vacuity or *qi* depression and blood stagnation, there is insufficient blood to moisten and nourish the heart and liver. This will result in vexation, agitation, irascibility, and breast distention.

Pulse:

A stringlike pulse.

Analysis

- The stringlike pulse is long, and feels like the string of a musical instrument.

Internal Static Blood Obstruction

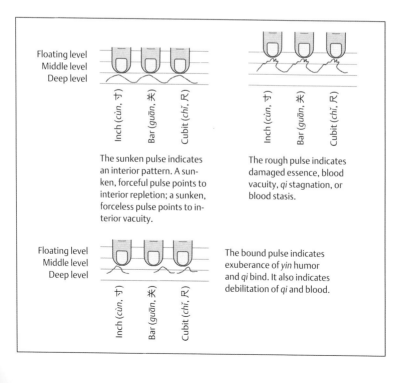

Floating level
Middle level
Deep level

Inch (*cùn*, 寸)   Bar (*guān*, 关)   Cubit (*chǐ*, 尺)

The sunken pulse indicates an interior pattern. A sunken, forceful pulse points to interior repletion; a sunken, forceless pulse points to interior vacuity.

Inch (*cùn*, 寸)   Bar (*guān*, 关)   Cubit (*chǐ*, 尺)

The rough pulse indicates damaged essence, blood vacuity, *qi* stagnation, or blood stasis.

Floating level
Middle level
Deep level

Inch (*cùn*, 寸)   Bar (*guān*, 关)   Cubit (*chǐ*, 尺)

The bound pulse indicates exuberance of *yin* humor and *qi* bind. It also indicates debilitation of *qi* and blood.

Signs and symptoms

Premenstrual or menstrual lower abdominal hardness and pain that refuses pressure, dark purple menstrual flow with stasis clots, pain relief after passage of the clots, a sooty-black facial complexion, encrusted skin (in severe cases), a purplish green-blue tongue with stasis macules, dark distended sublingual veins, thin white tongue fur, and a pulse that is sunken and rough, or sunken and bound.

Premenstrual or menstrual lower abdominal hardness and pain that refuses pressure:

Static blood collecting and stagnating in the body will, in severe cases, form a lump glomus (*pǐ kuài*, 痞塊), which blocks the movement of *qi* and blood. As a result, there is premenstrual or menstrual lower abdominal hardness and pain that refuses pressure.

Pain relief after passage of the clots:

When the blood clots are discharged, the level of blood stasis in the body will naturally decrease, resulting in relief of the pain.

Sooty-black facial complexion or, in severe cases, encrusted skin:

Blood stasis obstruction and stagnation cause inhibited movement of *qi* and blood, which makes it difficult for the fleshy exterior of the head and face to acquire moisture and nourishment. This produces a sooty-black facial complexion or encrusted skin.

Pulse:

A pulse that is sunken and rough, or sunken and bound.

Analysis

- The sunken pulse cannot be felt with light finger pressure. It is felt when heavy pressure is applied.
- The rough pulse is slow, thin, and short. It has a harsh onset and recession.
- The bound pulse is slow and sluggish, and pauses periodically at irregular intervals.

Blood Vacuity and Congealing Cold

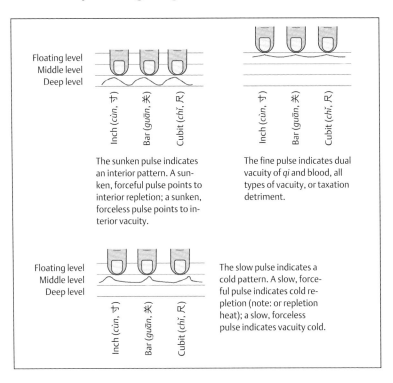

The sunken pulse indicates an interior pattern. A sunken, forceful pulse points to interior repletion; a sunken, forceless pulse points to interior vacuity.

The fine pulse indicates dual vacuity of *qi* and blood, all types of vacuity, or taxation detriment.

The slow pulse indicates a cold pattern. A slow, forceful pulse indicates cold repletion (note: or repletion heat); a slow, forceless pulse indicates vacuity cold.

Signs and symptoms

Premenstrual or menstrual lower abdominal pain that likes warmth and pressure, scant pale-colored menstrual flow, pain that is accompanied by cold or numb hands and feet, a pale tongue with white tongue fur, and a sunken, fine, and slow pulse.

Premenstrual or menstrual lower abdominal pain that likes warmth and pressure:

Women with blood vacuity constitutions who contract cold evil will have cold evil collecting and gathering in the stomach duct and abdomen. This will obstruct the normal movement of *qi* and blood, resulting in premenstrual or menstrual lower abdominal pain that likes warmth and pressure.

Pain that is accompanied by cold or numb hands and feet:

Blood vacuity leads to *yin* cold congealing and stagnating; as a result, the four limbs are deprived of warmth and nourishment, causing cold or numb hands and feet.

Scant, pale-colored menstrual flow:

If blood is vacuous, it is unable to fill the thoroughfare (*chōng*, 衝) and controlling (*rèn*, 任) vessels, leading to scant, pale-colored menstrual flow.

Pulse:

A sunken, fine, and slow pulse.

Analysis

- The sunken pulse cannot be felt with light finger pressure. It is felt when heavy pressure is applied.
- The fine pulse is thin (like a thread) yet clear.
- The slow pulse has a slow onset and recession. It beats three times per respiration.

Leukorrhea

Yang Vacuity with Exuberant Dampness

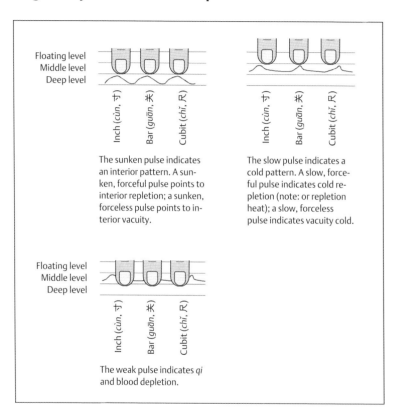

Floating level
Middle level
Deep level

Inch (*cùn*, 寸) Bar (*guān*, 关) Cubit (*chǐ*, 尺)

The sunken pulse indicates an interior pattern. A sunken, forceful pulse points to interior repletion; a sunken, forceless pulse points to interior vacuity.

Floating level
Middle level
Deep level

Inch (*cùn*, 寸) Bar (*guān*, 关) Cubit (*chǐ*, 尺)

The slow pulse indicates a cold pattern. A slow, forceful pulse indicates cold repletion (note: or repletion heat); a slow, forceless pulse indicates vacuity cold.

Floating level
Middle level
Deep level

Inch (*cùn*, 寸) Bar (*guān*, 关) Cubit (*chǐ*, 尺)

The weak pulse indicates *qi* and blood depletion.

Signs and symptoms

Incessant dribbling of thin white vaginal discharge that increases in quantity with exposure to cold, excruciating pain in the lumbus, cold pain in the lower abdomen, frequent long voidings of clear urine, sloppy diarrhea, a pale tongue with white, moist or glossy tongue fur, and a pulse that is sunken, slow, and weak.

Incessant dribbling of thin white vaginal discharge that increases in quantity with exposure to cold:
Kidney *yang* insufficiency leads to the internal generation of vacuity cold, which congeals and gathers in the lower burner. This causes failure of the girdling vessel (*dài mài*, 帶脈) to ensure retention and insecurity of the controlling vessel (*rèn mài*, 任脈), resulting in an incessant dribbling of thin white vaginal discharge that increases in quantity with exposure to cold.

Excruciating pain in the lumbus:
The lumbus is the house of the kidney; kidney vacuity causes an inability to transform and engender *qi* and blood, which leads to a depletion and inhibited movement of *qi* and blood. As a result, there is excruciating pain in the lumbus.

Cold pain in the lower abdomen:
Insufficiency of kidney *yang* leads to exuberant internal *yin* cold. When *yin* cold *qi* congeals and gathers in the lower burner, there is cold pain in the lower abdomen.

Frequent long voidings of clear urine:
Insufficiency of kidney *yang* causes impaired *qi* transformation in the urinary bladder, resulting in frequent long voidings of clear urine.

Sloppy diarrhea:
Depletion of kidney *yang* causes an inability of *yang qi* to move and transform water–damp. Water–damp then pours downward into the large intestine and impairs conveyance in the large intestine. This results in sloppy diarrhea.

Pulse:
A pulse that is sunken, slow, and weak.

Analysis

- The sunken pulse cannot be felt with light finger pressure. It is felt when heavy pressure is applied.
- The slow pulse has a slow onset and recession. It beats three times per respiration.
- The weak pulse is felt at the deep level. It is soft and forceless.

Exuberant Internal Damp–Heat

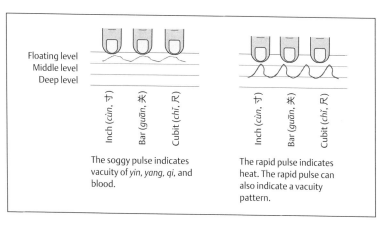

Floating level
Middle level
Deep level

Inch (*cùn*, 寸) Bar (*guān*, 关) Cubit (*chǐ*, 尺)

Inch (*cùn*, 寸) Bar (*guān*, 关) Cubit (*chǐ*, 尺)

The soggy pulse indicates vacuity of *yin, yang, qi,* and blood.

The rapid pulse indicates heat. The rapid pulse can also indicate a vacuity pattern.

Signs and symptoms

A sticky, slimy, fishy-smelling vaginal discharge of a yellow or yellow and white color, chest oppression, a slimy sensation in the mouth, torpid intake, continuous dull pain in the lower abdomen, short voidings of reddish urine, a red tongue with yellow slimy tongue fur, and a soggy and rapid pulse.

Sticky, slimy, fishy-smelling vaginal discharge of a yellow or yellow and white color:
Dampness evil is heavy and turbid by nature. The color white indicates dampness and the color yellow indicates heat. When dampness and heat evil fumigate and scorch the interior, damp turbidity congeals and gathers, giving rise to sticky, slimy, fish-smelling vaginal discharge of a yellow or yellow and white color.

Chest oppression and slimy sensation in the mouth:
Damp–heat collecting and stagnating in the chest and diaphragm blocks the up-bearing and downbearing of the *qi* dy-

namic and causes chest oppression. Dampness is, by nature, heavy and turbid; when damp turbidity overflows upward into the mouth, a slimy sensation is produced in the mouth.

Torpid intake:
Damp–heat collecting and gathering in the middle burner causes failure of the spleen to move and transform, resulting in reduced food intake.

Continuous dull pain in the lower abdomen:
Evil heat collects and stagnates in the lower burner. Dampness and heat contend with each other, bind together, and

linger there, causing continuous dull pain in the lower abdomen.

Short voidings of reddish urine:
Damp–heat evil collects and stagnates in the lower burner. The evil heat attempts to exit the body through the lower burner, causing short voidings of reddish urine.

Pulse:
A soggy and rapid pulse.

Analysis

- The soggy pulse is floating, thin and soft.
- The rapid pulse beats five or more times per respiration.

Menopausal Syndrome

Yin and *Yang* Vacuity Detriment

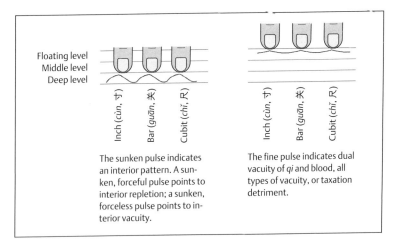

Floating level
Middle level
Deep level

Inch (*cùn*, 寸)   Bar (*guān*, 关)   Cubit (*chǐ*, 尺)

Inch (*cùn*, 寸)   Bar (*guān*, 关)   Cubit (*chǐ*, 尺)

The sunken pulse indicates an interior pattern. A sunken, forceful pulse points to interior repletion; a sunken, forceless pulse points to interior vacuity.

The fine pulse indicates dual vacuity of *qi* and blood, all types of vacuity, or taxation detriment.

Signs and symptoms

Perimenopausal fever and sweating, dizziness and tinnitus, vexation and agitation, insomnia, a limp, aching lumbus and knees, cold limbs, thin white tongue fur, and a sunken, fine pulse.

Perimenopausal fever and sweating:

Internal vacuity of *yin*, *yang*, *qi*, and blood gives rise to an internal generation of vacuity heat. The resulting insufficiency of defensive *yang* is unable to protect the fleshy exterior of the body, which leads to the inability of construction *yin* to guard the interior. This causes fever and sweating.

Limp, aching lumbus and knees with cold limbs:

Internal vacuity of *yin*, *yang*, *qi*, and blood leads to an insufficiency of kidney *qi*, which is then unable to fill and nourish the sinews and bones, producing a limp, aching lumbus and knees. In addition, *yang qi* depletion leads to impaired *qi* and blood production, which leads to an inability to warm the limbs, resulting in cold limbs.

Dizziness and tinnitus:

Insufficient kidney *qi* cannot fill and nourish the sea of marrow, causing dizziness and tinnitus.

Vexation, agitation and insomnia:

Insufficiency of liver blood leads to an internal generation of vacuity heat, which harasses the interior and causes failure of the ethereal soul (*hún*,) to keep to its abode. As a result, there is vexation and agitation. If there is lack of interaction between the heart spirit and kidney *yin* due to kidney *yin* depletion, there will also be insomnia.

Pulse:

A sunken, fine pulse.

Analysis

- The sunken pulse cannot be felt with light finger pressure. It is felt when heavy pressure is applied.
- The fine pulse is thin (like a thread) yet clear.

Liver and Kidney *Yin* Vacuity

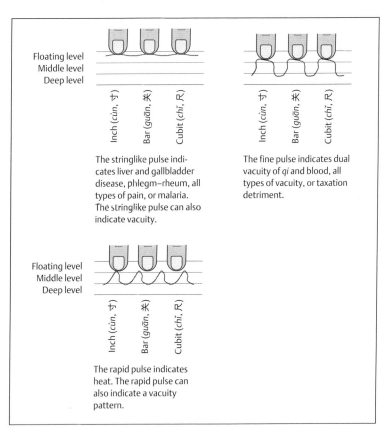

Floating level
Middle level
Deep level

Inch (cùn, 寸)   Bar (guān, 关)   Cubit (chǐ, 尺)

The stringlike pulse indicates liver and gallbladder disease, phlegm–rheum, all types of pain, or malaria. The stringlike pulse can also indicate vacuity.

Inch (cùn, 寸)   Bar (guān, 关)   Cubit (chǐ, 尺)

The fine pulse indicates dual vacuity of *qi* and blood, all types of vacuity, or taxation detriment.

Floating level
Middle level
Deep level

Inch (cùn, 寸)   Bar (guān, 关)   Cubit (chǐ, 尺)

The rapid pulse indicates heat. The rapid pulse can also indicate a vacuity pattern.

Signs and symptoms

Perimenopausal limp aching lumbus and knees, afternoon tidal fever, heat in the palms and soles, fullness and oppression in the chest and rib-side, vexation and agitation, insomnia, a bitter taste in the mouth, dry throat, irregular menstruation, scant and thin menstrual flow, a red tongue, scant tongue fur, and a pulse that is stringlike, fine, and rapid.

Perimenopausal limp, aching lumbus and knees:

During perimenopause, the prenatal *qi* (*xiān tiān qì*, 先天氣) of a woman with constitutional liver and kidney *yin* vacuity will be even more debilitated. Consequently, kidney *qi* is unable to fill the kidney and nourish the bones, thus producing a limp, aching lumbus and knees.

Afternoon tidal fever:

At noon, the body's *yang qi* starts to wane gradually, as *yin qi* grows. However, due to a depletion of constitutional *yin* humor, *yin* humor insufficiency leads to a prevalence of vacuity heat. This excessive vacuity heat penetrates outward into the fleshy exterior, giving rise to afternoon tidal fever.

Heat in the palms and soles:

Depletion of *yin* humor causes an internal generation of vacuity fire. Furthermore, *yin* vacuity leads to the inability of water to restrain fire; this results in fire heat thrusting outward into the four extremities, producing heat in the palms and soles.

Fullness and oppression in the chest and rib-side:

Impaired free coursing of the liver leads to inhibited diffusion and downbearing of the *qi* dynamic, while vacuity fire blocks chest *yang*. This combination results in fullness and oppression in the chest and rib-side.

Vexation, agitation and insomnia:

Internal generation of vacuity heat harasses and stirs the heart spirit, causing vexation and agitation. In addition, if there is a lack of interaction between the heart spirit and kidney *yin* due to depletion of kidney *yin*, there will also be insomnia.

Bitter taste in the mouth and dry throat:

A depletion of *yin* humor leads to internal generation of vacuity fire, which rises upward with liver and gallbladder *qi*, causing a bitter taste in the mouth and a dry throat.

Irregular menstruation with scant, thin menstrual flow:

During perimenopause, *qi* and blood insufficiency will result in debilitation of the thoroughfare (*chōng*, 衝) and controlling (*rèn*, 任) vessels. This causes irregular menstruation with a scant, thin menstrual flow.

Pulse:

A pulse that is stringlike, fine, and rapid.

Analysis

- The stringlike pulse is long, and feels like the string of a musical instrument.
- The fine pulse is thin (like a thread) yet clear.
- The rapid pulse beats five or more times per respiration.

4 *The Pulse Canon* (Mài Jīng, 脈經), Volume 8, written by Wáng Shū-Hé, Imperial Physician of the *Jìn* (晉) Dynasty

The Pulse Canon, written by Wáng Shū-Hé, is the first most comprehensive treatise on pulse theory in the history of Chinese medicine. It established the foundation of pulse theory over the last two thousand years. Consequently, anyone who is studying the pulse cannot do without knowledge of *The Pulse Canon*'s content. *The Pulse Canon* is divided into 10 volumes that separately discuss *yin–yang*, exterior–interior, the Three Positions and Nine Indicators, and the 24 pulses. The volumes also discuss *On Cold Damage* (*Shāng Hán Lùn*, 傷寒論) and the pulse, signs, and treatment of various diseases. The canon serves to show the accumulated experience on pulse theory of that time period, making it an indispensable text. On the following pages you will find discussions on several chapters of the canon.

■ Chapter 1: Discussion of the Pulse and Signs of Sudden Death-like Reversal

Key points emphasized

- Discusses the pulse manifestation and signs of sudden death-like reversal (sudden fainting).
- The pulse manifestation is sunken, large, and slippery. A sunken and large pulse indicates repletion evil in the interior. A slippery pulse indicates stagnation of the *qi* dynamic. In short, this pulse manifestation indicates the repletion evil and the *qi* dynamic contending with each other and binding together.
- The disease pattern of sudden fainting: If the evil *qi* enters the viscera, the patient will die; if the evil *qi* enters the bowels, the disease condition will improve with ease.

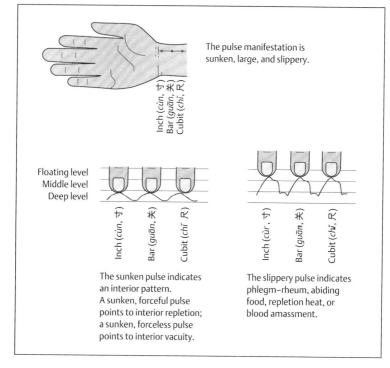

The pulse manifestation is sunken, large, and slippery.

Floating level
Middle level
Deep level

Inch (cùn, 寸)
Bar (guān, 关)
Cubit (chǐ, 尺)

The sunken pulse indicates an interior pattern.
A sunken, forceful pulse points to interior repletion; a sunken, forceless pulse points to interior vacuity.

The slippery pulse indicates phlegm–rheum, abiding food, repletion heat, or blood amassment.

– If, during sudden fainting, the lips and mouth are green-blue (*qīng*, 青) or purple, and the body is icy-cold, this is evil *qi* entering the viscera, a disease condition that is critical. If the entire body is warm and harmonious with spontaneous sweating, this is evil *qi* entering the bowels, a disease condition that can easily improve.

Evil *qi* entering the viscera:
If, during sudden fainting, the lips and mouth are green-blue (*qīng*, 青) or purple and the body is icy cold, this is evil *qi* entering the viscera, a disease condition that is critical.

Evil *qi* entering the bowels:
If the entire body is warm and harmonious with spontaneous sweating, this represents evil *qi* entering the bowels, a disease condition that can easily improve.

▪ Chapter 2: Discussion of the Pulse and Signs of Tetany, Dampness, and Thermoplegia

Key points emphasized

- Discusses the pulse manifestation, signs, and medicinal treatment of tetany, dampness, and thermoplegia.
- A wind–cold-induced greater *yang* exterior repletion pattern manifesting as fever, absence of sweating, and aversion to cold is called hard tetany (*gāng jìng*, 剛痙).
- A wind–cold-induced greater *yang* exterior vacuity pattern manifesting as fever, sweating, and absence of aversion to cold is called soft tetany (*róu jìng*, 柔痙).

Hard tetany:
Manifests as fever, absence of sweating, and aversion to cold.

Soft tetany:
Manifests as fever, sweating, and absence of aversion to cold.

In the case of fever in greater *yang* disease, the pulse manifestation should be floating; if, conversely, the pulse manifestation is sunken and fine, this indicates tetany of the right *qi* insufficiency (exuberant evil and vacuous right) pattern.

Tetany:
Insufficiency of right *qi* (exuberant evil and vacuous right) manifests with a sunken and fine pulse.

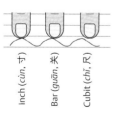

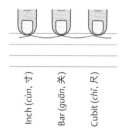

Floating level
Middle level
Deep level

Inch (*cùn*, 寸)
Bar (*guān*, 关)
Cubit (*chǐ*, 尺)

Inch (*cùn*, 寸)
Bar (*guān*, 关)
Cubit (*chǐ*, 尺)

The sunken pulse indicates an interior pattern.
A sunken, forceful pulse points to interior repletion; a sunken, forceless pulse points to interior vacuity.

The fine pulse indicates dual vacuity of *qi* and blood, all types of vacuity, or taxation detriment.

> *The exterior pattern of greater* yang *disease should not be treated with excessive diaphoresis.*

Excessive sweating will cause the body fluids to be consumed and the sinews to be deprived of nourishment, giving rise to tetany.

Those who suffer from greater *yang* disease exterior pattern present with fever and cold feet, a red face, aversion to cold, hypertonicity and rigidity of the neck and nape, and a limited range of head motion; this is called tetany.

A greater *yang* exterior repletion pattern manifests as absence of sweating, reduced urination (contrary to what is expected), a counterflow upsurge of *qi* to the chest region, and a clenched jaw with inability to open the mouth to speak. These are the signs of impending hard tetany; use Pueraria Decoction (*Gé Gēn Tāng*, 葛根湯) to treat this.

During the onset of hard tetany, the patient presents with fullness and oppression in the chest region, a clenched jaw, noisy grinding of the teeth, arching of the back with an inability to lie in bed, and spasm and hypertonicity of the legs; one can use Major *Qi*-Coordinating Decoction (*Dà Chéng Qì Tāng*, 大承氣湯) to treat this.

If, in tetany, the pulse becomes sunken and hidden, this suggests no improvement of the disease condition.

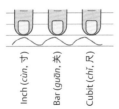

Floating level
Middle level
Deep level

Inch (*cùn*, 寸)   Bar (*guān*, 关)   Cubit (*chǐ*, 尺)

The sunken pulse indicates an interior pattern.
A sunken, forceful pulse points to interior repletion; a sunken, forceless pulse points to interior vacuity.

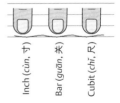

Inch (*cùn*, 寸)   Bar (*guān*, 关)   Cubit (*chǐ*, 尺)

The hidden pulse indicates evil block, reversal pattern (*jué zhèng*, 厥證), or pain.

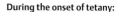

During the onset of tetany:
The pulse is stringlike and forceful.

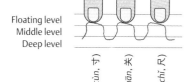

Floating level
Middle level
Deep level

Inch (*cùn*, 寸)
Bar (*guān*, 关)
Cubit (*chǐ*, 尺)

The stringlike pulse indicates liver and gallbladder disease, phlegm–rheum, all types of pain, or malaria. The stringlike pulse can also indicate vacuity.

If, in tetany, the pulse becomes slippery and soft after sweating is induced, and is accompanied by a normal tongue, and there is no longer a sunken depression in the abdominal region from arched-back rigidity, this indicates improvement of the disease condition. If there is no other change in the pulse manifestation, but the pulse becomes sunken and hidden, this indicates no improvement of the disease condition.

During the onset of tetany, the quality of the pulse from the inch (*cùn*) position to the cubit (*chǐ*) position will be stringlike and forceful.

The usual pulse manifestation (from the inch position to the cubit position) of tetany is sunken, hidden, and tight, and feels hard.

> *For those suffering from invasion of wind evil,* yin *humor will be consumed if draining precipitation is used erroneously.*

If draining precipitation (*xiè xià fǎ*, 瀉下法) is used erroneously for those suffering from invasion of wind evil, *yin* humor will be consumed and the sinews will be deprived of nourishment, giving rise to tetany. If this condition is further treated with strong diaphoresis, it will lead to severe hypertonicity of the body.

The symptoms of greater *yang* disease exterior pattern are fever, sweating, aversion to wind, and stiffness and pain in the head and nape of the neck; if they are accompanied by rigidity of the body, neck, and nape with a sunken, slow pulse (when it should be floating), the condition is tetany. Use Trichosanthes and Cinnamon Twig Decoction (*Guā Lóu Guì Zhī Tāng*, 栝蔞桂枝湯) to treat it.

> *If a patient with tetany concurrently suffers from sores, the disease condition will worsen and become difficult to treat.*

If a patient with tetany already suffers from pre-existing sores (*chuāng yáng bìng*, 瘡瘍病), liquid (*jīn*, 津) and blood is depleted early on due to the festering and maceration of the sores, there will, with the addition of tetany, be desiccation of blood and damage to liquid. The disease condition will worsen and become difficult to treat.

A person suffering from sores who concurrently has generalized body pain from greater *yang* disease should not be treated with diaphoresis, or body fluids will be consumed and tetany will develop.

If greater *yang* disease presents with joint pain, vexation, and agitation, and a sunken, moderate pulse, this is due to dampness evil collecting and stagnating to form impediment pattern (*hì zhèng*, 痹證).

If there is pain of the whole body and fever that worsens at dusk, this is wind–damp. It is caused by exposure to wind and dampness while sweating.

A person suffering from damp impediment may present with pain of the whole body, fever, and a dark, smoky-yellow skin color.

Impediment:
Dampness evil collects and stagnates to form an impediment pattern. The pulse is sunken and moderate.

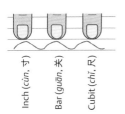
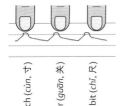

Floating level
Middle level
Deep level

Inch (*cùn*, 寸) Bar (*guān*, 关) Cubit (*chǐ*, 尺)

Inch (*cùn*, 寸) Bar (*guān*, 关) Cubit (*chǐ*, 尺)

The sunken pulse indicates an interior pattern.
A sunken, forceful pulse points to interior repletion; a sunken, forceless pulse points to interior vacuity.

The moderate pulse indicates dampness or spleen vacuity.

> *If one erroneously uses draining precipitation to treat a person suffering from dampness disease, there will be hiccough or fullness and oppression in the chest and diaphragm.*

Those suffering from dampness disease have a tendency to sweat in the head region, back stiffness, and aversion to cold with a desire to stay under the covers for warmth. If one erroneously uses draining precipitation to treat this condition, there will be hiccough or fullness and oppression in the chest and diaphragm. Inhibited urination and moist, white glossy tongue fur are due to heat in the cinnabar field (*dān tián*, 丹田) and cold in the chest region and upper burner, resulting in thirst with no desire to drink and a dry mouth. This is a result of water–damp causing internal obstruction, and evil heat congestion.

Because heat in the cinnabar field and cold in the chest region and upper burner results in thirst with no desire to drink and a dry mouth, mistreating a person suffering from dampness disease by using draining precipitation will produce sweating in the forehead, slight panting, and inhibited urination; this is reversal collapse of *yin* and *yang*, a fatal sign. If there is incessant clear-food diarrhea, this indicates exhaustion of both *yin* and *yang*, which is also a fatal sign.

> ***Question:*** *When wind and dampness invade the body, there is generalized body pain, which should be treated with diaphoresis. It is said that diaphoresis can be used to treat a person exposed to overcast and rainy weather. Conversely, however, the disease condition does not improve from this treatment. What is the cause of this?*
>
> ***Answer:*** *This is because although strong diaphoresis dispels and scatters wind evil, it cannot eliminate the dampness evil. As a result, the patient is unable to fully recover from the disease condition.*
>
> *To treat dampness disease, one should administer mild diaphoresis to restore the unimpeded flow of the construction (*yíng*, 營) and defense (*wèi*, 衛). Only then can the wind-damp evil be successfully eliminated.*

> *Those suffering from dampness disease should not be treated with fire-attacking methods or excessive diaphoresis.*

Those suffering from dampness disease presenting with generalized body pains, vexation, and agitation, can be treated with Ephedra Decoction (*Má Huáng Tāng*, 麻黃湯) plus four taels (*liǎng*, 兩) of *bái zhú* (Atractylodis Macrocephalae Rhizoma); this will promote mild sweating. One should not use a fire-attacking method or excessive diaphoresis.

In wind-damp disease, there is generalized body heaviness with a floating pulse, and sweating accompanied by aversion to wind; one may use Fangji Decoction (*Fáng Jǐ Tāng*, 防己湯) to treat this.

If there is panting, headache, nasal congestion with vexation, a large pulse, a normal diet, and stomach and intestinal harmony, this signifies no change in the disease state. If cold–damp evil invades the head region and gives rise to nasal congestion, this can be treated by stuffing the nose with medicinals to drain liquid from the upper burner, thereby allowing the lung *qi* to flow freely.

If cold damage exterior pattern is unresolved for eight or nine days, wind and dampness will contend with each other and accumulate, giving rise to pain of the whole body, an inability to turn over, absence of vomiting, absence of thirst, and a pulse that is floating, vacuous, and rough. At this time, the evil *qi* has not yet entered the interior. Use Cinnamon Twig and Aconite Decoction (*Guì Zhī Fù Zǐ Tāng*, 桂枝附子湯) to treat this condition. If the patient has dry stools and uninhibited urination, Atractylodes and Aconite Decoction (*Bái Zhú Fù Zǐ Tāng*, 白术附子湯) can be used as treatment.

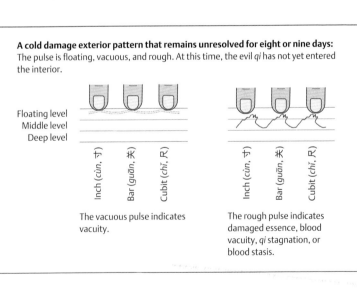

A cold damage exterior pattern that remains unresolved for eight or nine days: The pulse is floating, vacuous, and rough. At this time, the evil *qi* has not yet entered the interior.

Floating level
Middle level
Deep level

Inch (cùn, 寸)   Bar (guān, 关)   Cubit (chǐ, 尺)

Inch (cùn, 寸)   Bar (guān, 关)   Cubit (chǐ, 尺)

The vacuous pulse indicates vacuity.

The rough pulse indicates damaged essence, blood vacuity, *qi* stagnation, or blood stasis.

Chapter 3: Discussion of the Pulse and Signs of *Yang* Toxin, *Yin* Toxin, Lily Disease, and Fox-Creeper Disease

Key points emphasized

– Discusses the pulse manifestation, signs, and medicinal treatment of *yin* and *yang* toxin, lily disease, and fox-creeper disease.

– *Yang* toxin disease due to contraction of epidemic toxin is characterized by body heaviness, lumbus and back pain, vexation and oppression, manic raving and nonsensical talk, walking about aimlessly, behaving as if one has seen a ghost, or vomiting of blood and diarrhea, a pulse that is floating, large, and rapid, red macules on the face, sore throat, and vomiting of pus and blood.

– If the right *qi* of a patient affected by *yang* toxin disease has not yet been weakened, a cure is still possible within five days. If, after the seventh day, there is exuberant *yang* toxin with exhaustion of right *qi*, a cure is difficult.

– In only one or two days, cold damage disease can transmute into *yang* toxin pattern. Patients who have been mistreated with medicinals that induce emesis or precipitation can also develop *yang* toxin pattern. Cimicifuga Decoction (*Shēng Má Tāng*, 升麻湯) can be used to treat this condition.

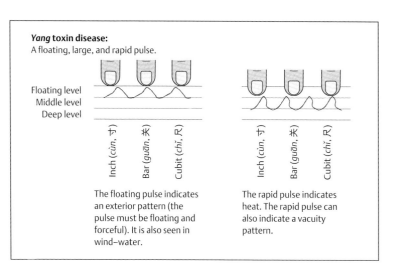

Yang **toxin disease:**
A floating, large, and rapid pulse.

Floating level
Middle level
Deep level

Inch (*cùn*, 寸) Bar (*guān*, 关) Cubit (*chǐ*, 尺)

Inch (*cùn*, 寸) Bar (*guān*, 关) Cubit (*chǐ*, 尺)

The floating pulse indicates an exterior pattern (the pulse must be floating and forceful). It is also seen in wind–water.

The rapid pulse indicates heat. The rapid pulse can also indicate a vacuity pattern.

> *Both cold damage disease and the erroneous administration of medicinals that induce emesis or precipitation can lead to the development of* yang *toxin pattern.*

Yin toxin disease due to the contraction of epidemic toxin is characterized by body heaviness, back rigidity, gripping pain in the abdomen, and sore throat. If the epidemic toxin attacks the heart, there will be hard glomus below the heart, shortness of breath, retching, a dark facial complexion, green-blue or purple

---

Yin toxin disease:
A sunken, fine, tight, and rapid pulse.

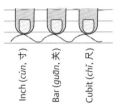

Floating level
Middle level
Deep level

Inch (cùn, 寸)
Bar (guān, 关)
Cubit (chǐ, 尺)

The sunken pulse indicates an interior pattern.
A sunken, forceful pulse points to interior repletion; a sunken, forceless pulse points to interior vacuity.

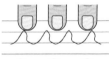

Inch (cùn, 寸)
Bar (guān, 关)
Cubit (chǐ, 尺)

The fine pulse indicates dual vacuity of *qi* and blood, all types of vacuity, or taxation detriment.

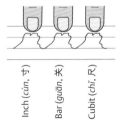

Floating level
Middle level
Deep level

Inch (cùn, 寸)
Bar (guān, 关)
Cubit (chǐ, 尺)

The tight pulse indicates cold, pain, or abiding food.

Inch (cùn, 寸)
Bar (guān, 关)
Cubit (chǐ, 尺)

The rapid pulse indicates heat. The rapid pulse can also indicate a vacuity pattern.

lips, icy-cold hands and feet, generalized body pain (as if due to physical injury), and a pulse that is sunken, fine, tight, and rapid.

If the patient's right *qi* has not yet been exhausted, a cure is possible within five days. If, after the seventh day, there is exuberant *yin* toxin with right *qi* exhaustion, a cure is difficult.

In only 1 or 2 days, cold damage disease can transmute into *yin* toxin pattern. Patients who have received erroneous medicinal treatment for 6 or 7 to 10 days can also develop *yin* toxin pattern. Licorice Decoction (*Gān Cǎo Tāng*, 甘草湯) can be used to treat this condition.

> *Both cold damage disease and the erroneous administration of vomit-inducing or precipitating medicinals can lead to the development of* yin *toxin pattern.*

Those who suffer from lily disease often exhibit taciturnity, desire to sleep but inability to sleep, desire to walk but inability to do so, desire to eat but being unable to eat, occasional good appetite and occasional aversion to the smell of food and beverages, a subjective sensation of cold, subjective fever, a bitter taste in the mouth upon rising in the morning, and yellow or reddish urine. These patients appear strong and healthy on the surface, yet the pulse is faint and rapid. This is because lily disease primarily affects the heart and lung (and thus affects the blood and vessels), and it should be treated according to the different signs.

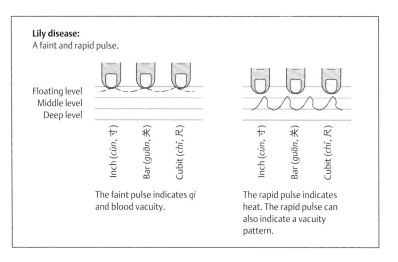

Lily disease:
A faint and rapid pulse.

Floating level
Middle level
Deep level

Inch (*cùn*, 寸)   Bar (*guān*, 关)   Cubit (*chǐ*, 尺)

Inch (*cùn*, 寸)   Bar (*guān*, 关)   Cubit (*chǐ*, 尺)

The faint pulse indicates *qi* and blood vacuity.

The rapid pulse indicates heat. The rapid pulse can also indicate a vacuity pattern.

If lily disease manifests as a *yin* pattern, the treatment should involve supplementation of *yang*. If lily disease manifests as a *yang* pattern, it is appropriate to employ nourishment of *yin* as the treatment. If the *yang* pattern is treated with supplementation of *yang* in conjunction with diaphoresis, there will be double injury to the *yin* humor, thus rendering the disease condition more difficult to recover from.

> *Fox-creeper disease is caused by damp–heat toxic evil invasion leading to damp-heat brewing internally.*

Those who suffer from fox-creeper disease present with aversion to cold, fever, a resemblance of cold damage pattern, devitalized essence–spirit with sleepiness but an inability to close the eyes and sleep, and fidgetiness while lying down. This condition is caused by an invasion of damp–heat toxic evil, leading to damp–heat brewing internally. If erosions form in the throat, the condition is called creeper disease (*huò bìng*, 惑病). If erosions form on the anterior and posterior *yin* (genitals and anus), the condition is called fox disease (*hú bìng*, 狐病).

Patients with fox-creeper disease have not only no appetite, but also an aversion to the smell of food. The facial complexion can be red, white, or black. If damp–heat toxic evil gives rise to erosions in the throat, it will cause the voice to be hoarse. If damp–heat toxic evil gives rise to erosions in the two *yin* (anal and genital orifices), the throat will be dry.

When the upper region (throat) is eroded, one may treat this with Heart-Draining Decoction (*Xiè Xīn Tāng*, 瀉心湯). When the lower *yin* regions are

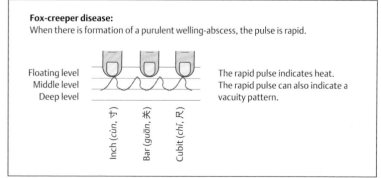

Fox-creeper disease:
When there is formation of a purulent welling-abscess, the pulse is rapid.

Floating level
Middle level
Deep level

Inch (cùn, 寸) Bar (guān, 关) Cubit (chǐ, 尺)

The rapid pulse indicates heat.
The rapid pulse can also indicate a vacuity pattern.

eroded, use Flavescent Sophora Decoction (*Kǔ Shēn Tāng*, 苦參湯) as a steam-wash. When the anus is eroded, treat this by fumigating the affected area with *xióng huáng* (Realgar).

When a purulent welling-abscess forms in fox-creeper disease, it manifests with a rapid pulse, absence of fever, vexation and oppression, devitalized essence–spirit, sleepiness, and sweating. Within three or four days of the onset of this disease, the eyes become as red as those of a turtledove; by the seventh or eighth day, a yellowish-black color appears at the inner and outer corners of the eyes, at which time there is toxic evil binding and gathering in the head and eyes. As the spleen and stomach are mildly affected, the patient's appetite is normal. Rice Bean and Chinese Angelica Decoction (*Chì Xiǎo Dòu Dāng Guī Tāng*, 赤小豆當歸湯) should be the chosen formula.

◼ Chapter 4: Discussion of the Pulse and Signs of Sudden Turmoil and Cramps

Key points emphasized

– Discusses the pulse manifestation and signs of sudden turmoil (*huò luàn*, 霍亂) and cramps.

> *Question: What symptoms appear in sudden turmoil?*
>
> *Answer: Simultaneous vomiting and diarrhea is known as sudden turmoil.*
>
> *Question: If vomiting and diarrhea emerge several days after a patient experiences fever, headache, generalized pain, and aversion to cold, what is this disease?*
>
> *Answer: This is sudden turmoil. In sudden turmoil, after vomiting and diarrhea cease, there will (again) be fever. If the pattern is only that of cold damage, the pulse should be floating and tight; however, the pulse is faint and rough. This is because the person with sudden turmoil simultaneously contracts cold evil; four or five days later, the disease evil enters the yin channels, resulting in vomiting and diarrhea.*
>
> *Patients who suffer from cramp disease experience hypertonicity of the sinews in the arms and legs. The pulse is faint and stringlike from the inch (cùn) to the cubit (chǐ) positions. In severe cases, there is pain extending from the gastrocnemius muscle to the lower abdomen. Use White Chicken's Dropping Powder (Jī Shǐ Bái Sǎn, 雞屎白散) to treat this condition.*

In patients with sudden turmoil who simultaneously contract cold evil, the pulse is faint and rough.

Floating level
Middle level
Deep level

Inch (cùn, 寸)   Bar (guān, 关)   Cubit (chǐ, 尺)

Inch (cùn, 寸)   Bar (guān, 关)   Cubit (chǐ, 尺)

The faint pulse indicates *qi* and blood vacuity.

The rough pulse indicates damaged essence, blood vacuity, *qi* stagnation, or blood stasis.

■ Chapter 5: Discussion of the Pulse and Signs of Wind Strike and Joint-running Wind

Key points emphasized

– Discusses the pulse, signs, and treatment of joint-running wind.
– Disease patterns caused by wind strike (*zhòng fēng*, 中風) usually manifest as loss of mobility in one side of the body or loss of mobility in the upper extremity of either side of the body. This is impediment pattern due to *qi* and blood stasis obstruction, and the pulse should be faint and rapid.
– A headache with a slippery pulse is externally contracted wind strike, and should be accompanied by exterior symptoms. Wind strike from internal damage should manifest with a vacuous and weak pulse.

A tight pulse indicates wind–cold strike; a floating pulse indicates interior vacuity.

As for the floating and tight pulse manifestation, the tight pulse indicates wind–cold strike, and the floating pulse indicates interior vacuity. Vacuity and cold evil contend with each other and bind together, and the disease evil collects and stagnates in the skin. The floating pulse indicates *qi* and blood deple-

Wind strike causing impediment pattern of the *qi* and blood stasis obstruction type presents with a faint and rapid pulse.

Floating level
Middle level
Deep level

Inch (*cùn*, 寸)
Bar (*guān*, 关)
Cubit (*chǐ*, 尺)

Inch (*cùn*, 寸)
Bar (*guān*, 关)
Cubit (*chǐ*, 尺)

The faint pulse indicates *qi* and blood vacuity.

The rapid pulse indicates heat. The rapid pulse can also indicate a vacuity pattern.

tion; if *qi* and blood are depleted, the network vessels are empty and unable to fight (disease) evil. As a result, the evil *qi* cannot be discharged from the body, but instead collects and stagnates in the left or right side of the body. The side of the body affected by the evil will present with symptoms of flaccidity due to the resulting blockage in the network vessels. The normal, unaffected side of the body will present with hypertonicity (contrary to what is expected). The healthy side of the body will pull on the affected side, causing one-sided deviation of the eyes and mouth and loss of mobility.

The side of the body affected by the evil will present with symptoms of flaccidity due to the resulting blockage in the network vessels. The normal, unaffected side of the body will present with hypertonicity (contrary to what is expected).

If the disease evil enters the network vessels, the construction *qi* will be unable to nourish the fleshy exterior, and there will be numbness of the skin and flesh.

If the disease evil is lodged in the channels, *qi* and blood will be unable to nourish the limbs, and there will be heaviness of the limbs with an inability to lift them.

If the disease evil enters the bowels, there will be clouding loss of consciousness.

If the disease evil enters the viscera, there will be loss of speech and drooling from the corners of the mouth.

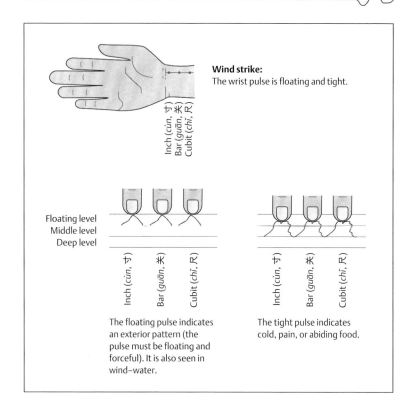

Wind strike:
The wrist pulse is floating and tight.

Floating level
Middle level
Deep level

Inch (cùn, 寸) Bar (guān, 关) Cubit (chǐ, 尺)

Inch (cùn, 寸) Bar (guān, 关) Cubit (chǐ, 尺)

The floating pulse indicates an exterior pattern (the pulse must be floating and forceful). It is also seen in wind–water.

The tight pulse indicates cold, pain, or abiding food.

A slow pulse is attributed to cold. A moderate pulse stands for vacuity.

As for the emergence of a slow and moderate pulse manifestation at the wrist, a slow pulse is attributed to cold, and a moderate pulse stands for vacuity. Depletion of construction and *yin* indicates blood collapse, and cold from vacuity of defense *qi* easily gives rise to wind strike.

If the disease evil affects the channels, there will be generalized itching and dormant papules on the skin. If the heart *qi* is insufficient and is affected by the disease evil, fullness and oppression of the chest and diaphragm and shortness of breath will arise.

The instep *yang* pulse is an indicator of stomach *qi*. If the instep *yang* pulse is floating and slippery, the slippery pulse stands for intense stomach heat, and

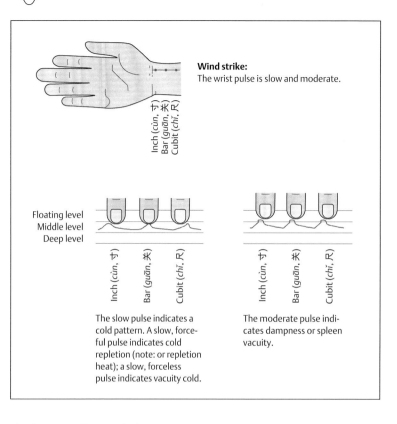

Wind strike:
The wrist pulse is slow and moderate.

Inch (cùn, 寸)
Bar (guān, 关)
Cubit (chǐ, 尺)

Floating level
Middle level
Deep level

Inch (cùn, 寸)
Bar (guān, 关)
Cubit (chǐ, 尺)

Inch (cùn, 寸)
Bar (guān, 关)
Cubit (chǐ, 尺)

The slow pulse indicates a cold pattern. A slow, forceful pulse indicates cold repletion (note: or repletion heat); a slow, forceless pulse indicates vacuity cold.

The moderate pulse indicates dampness or spleen vacuity.

the floating pulse stands for an exterior pattern; hence there is spontaneous sweating.

> *The instep* yang *pulse is an indicator of stomach* qi. *The lesser* yin *pulse is an indicator of the heart and kidney pulses.*

The lesser *yin* pulse is an indicator of the heart and kidney pulses. If the lesser *yin* pulse is floating and weak, the weak pulse indicates insufficiency of *yin* and blood, and the floating pulse indicates an exterior pattern. Evil *qi* and blood contend with each other and bind together, causing obstruction in the channels and depriving the sinews and bones of nourishment. This results in severe pain in the interstices of the flesh.

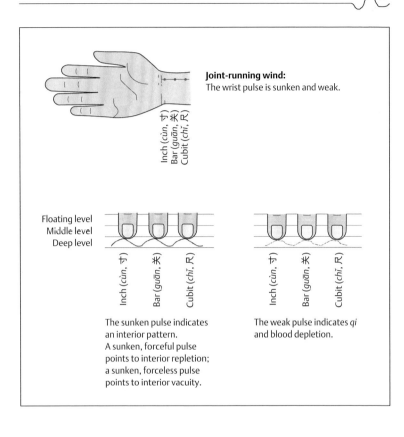

Joint-running wind:
The wrist pulse is sunken and weak.

Inch (cùn, 寸)
Bar (guān, 关)
Cubit (chǐ, 尺)

Floating level
Middle level
Deep level

Inch (cùn, 寸)
Bar (guān, 关)
Cubit (chǐ, 尺)

Inch (cùn, 寸)
Bar (guān, 关)
Cubit (chǐ, 尺)

The sunken pulse indicates
an interior pattern.
A sunken, forceful pulse
points to interior repletion;
a sunken, forceless pulse
points to interior vacuity.

The weak pulse indicates *qi*
and blood depletion.

If an obese person presents with a rough, small, and forceless pulse manifestation, a tendency towards shortness of breath, profuse sweating, and joint pain with inability to bend and stretch, this is due to exposure to wind evil after sweating from drinking alcohol; the wind and dampness contend with each other and bind together to cause this.

As for the sunken and weak pulse manifestation, the sunken quality is attributed to interior disease and indicates kidney *qi* insufficiency; the kidney governs the bones. The weak quality indicates liver blood insufficiency; the liver governs the sinews. Liver and kidney insufficiency is the cause of joint-running wind.

Excessive consumption of sour food damages the liver; if the liver is damaged, the sinews are damaged and become flaccid and useless. This results in loss of voluntary movement, and is known as sluggishness.

Excessive consumption of salty food damages the kidney; if the kidney is damaged, the bones are weakened, and the marrow desiccated. As a result, the patient is thin and weak, and unable to stand or walk. This is called desiccation.

> *Joint-running wind: If there is liver and kidney damage, and the patient is further exposed to external evil, the disease evil will gather and produce heat, thereby giving rise to joint-running wind.*

Liver and kidney damage results in exhaustion of construction–blood and defense *qi*, failure of the triple burner to move *qi* and blood, and lack of nourishment in the four limbs. As a result, there is emaciation with swelling of the lower legs and feet, yellow sweating, and a sensation of cold in the lower legs and feet.

If further exposed to external evil, the disease evil will gather and produce heat, thereby giving rise to joint-running wind. Patients with joint-running wind experience joint pain and a loss of voluntary bending and stretching. Aconite Main Tuber Decoction (*Wū Tóu Tāng*, 烏頭湯) can be used to treat this condition.

If patients with joint-running wind have pain in the joints of every limb, gradual emaciation, swelling of the feet as if they are about to be separated from the body, cloudiness and dizziness of the head and eyes, shortness of breath, and counterflow ascent of stomach *qi* with a desire to vomit, one may treat this with Cinnamon Twig, Peony, and Anemarrhena Decoction (*Guì Zhī Sháo Yào Zhī Mǔ Tāng*, 桂枝芍藥知母湯).

■ Chapter 6: Discussion of the Pulse and Signs of Blood Impediment and Vacuity Taxation

Key points emphasized

– Discusses the signs, pulse manifestation, and treatment of blood impediment and vacuity taxation.

> **Question:** *How is blood impediment acquired?*
> **Answer:** *People of high social status are well nourished with strong muscles but tend to have frail sinews and bones. They may also suffer from sweating during fatigue, tossing and turning during sleep, and difficulty falling asleep. If combined with wind–cold invasion, blood*

impediment can easily arise. On the surface, blood impediment seems to resemble wind strike; however, the overall pulse manifestation of blood impediment is faint and rough, and the bar (guān) position is small and tight. Using acupuncture to guide the yang qi and harmonize the blood vessels to dispel the cold and tight qi will produce a cure.

Note: *The* qi *and blood stasis obstruction (of an impediment pattern) caused by wind strike reveals a faint and rapid pulse manifestation; this is different from the pulse manifestation of blood impediment.*

In patients with blood impediment, *yin* and *yang* are debilitated. The bar (*guān*) position of the wrist pulse is faint and weak, while the cubit (*chǐ*) position is small and tight. There is numbness of the muscles. This pattern is similar to that of wind impediment. Use Astragalus and Cinnamon Twig Five Agents Decoction (*Huáng Qí Guì Zhī Wǔ Wù Tāng*, 黃耆桂枝五物湯) to treat this.

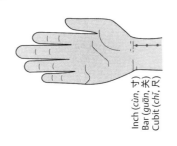

The overall pulse manifestation of blood impediment is faint and rough, and the bar (*guān*) position is faint and tight.

Inch (*cùn*, 寸)
Bar (*guān*, 关)
Cubit (*chǐ*, 尺)

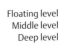

Floating level
Middle level
Deep level

Inch (*cùn*, 寸)
Bar (*guān*, 关)
Cubit (*chǐ*, 尺)

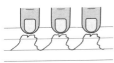

Inch (*cùn*, 寸)
Bar (*guān*, 关)
Cubit (*chǐ*, 尺)

The rough pulse indicates damaged essence, blood vacuity, *qi* stagnation, or blood stasis.

The tight pulse indicates cold, pain, or abiding food.

Vacuity taxation disease:
The pulse manifestation is large and forceless.

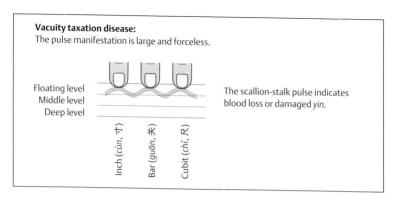

Floating level
Middle level
Deep level

Inch (cùn, 寸)
Bar (guān, 关)
Cubit (chǐ, 尺)

The scallion-stalk pulse indicates blood loss or damaged *yin*.

Some men, on the surface, seem as if they have no unusual disease pattern, but their pulse manifestations are large and forceless; this indicates floating of *yang* due to *yin* vacuity, which is a vacuity taxation disease. If the pulse manifestation is extremely vacuous, this indicates vacuity taxation from internal damage of essential *qi*.

> In vacuity taxation disease, the pulse manifestation is large and forceless; this is yang floating outward due to yin vacuity.

Men who suffer from vacuity taxation disease have a large and forceless pulse manifestation. This is *yang* floating outward due to *yin* vacuity. *Yin* vacuity produces internal heat, which gives rise to vexing heat in the palms. In the spring and summer, there is exuberance of heat, which will cause the disease condition to worsen. In the autumn, *yang qi* hides in the interior of the body, and therefore the disease condition will be mild. Internal exuberance of *yin* cold causes insecurity of the essence gate (resulting in spontaneous seminal emission), pain and emaciation of both legs with difficulty walking, and lesser abdominal vacuity fullness.

When a person reaches 50–60 years of age, the pulse manifestation becomes floating, large, and forceless. In addition, there is numbness of the spine and back due to blood impediment, rumbling intestines, and hard nodules in the armpits or sides of the neck. This is a result of vacuity taxation disease due to taxation damage.

> *A vacuous, weak, faint, and fine pulse indicates a tendency for night sweating.*

A vacuous, weak, faint, and fine pulse in men that seem to have no unusual disease pattern on the surface indicates a tendency toward night sweating.

A lusterless complexion in men indicates thirst and excessive loss of blood. If there is hasty, rapid breathing with palpitations, and a pulse that is floating, large, and forceless, the cause is interior vacuity.

A vacuous, sunken, and stringlike pulse in men who have no symptoms of externally contracted cold or heat, yet exhibit shortness of breath, abdominal pain, inhibited urination, a somber white facial complexion, clouded flowery vision, a tendency for nosebleeds, and lower abdominal distention and fullness indicates dual vacuity of *qi* and blood from vacuity taxation.

> *A vacuous, sunken, and stringlike pulse manifestation in men reveals dual vacuity of qi and blood from vacuity taxation.*

A faint, weak, and rough pulse manifestation in men indicates infertility; this is a result of insufficiency of essential *qi*, which leads to clear, thin, and icy-cold semen.

Seminal emission:
A faint, weak, and rough pulse manifestation in men indicates infertility.

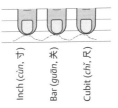
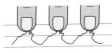

Floating level
Middle level
Deep level

Inch (cùn, 寸)   Bar (guān, 关)   Cubit (chǐ, 尺)

Inch (cùn, 寸)   Bar (guān, 关)   Cubit (chǐ, 尺)

The weak pulse indicates *qi* and blood depletion.

The rough pulse indicates damaged essence, blood vacuity, *qi* stagnation, or blood stasis.

Deserting *qi*:
A sunken, small, and slow pulse indicates spleen and kidney debilitation.

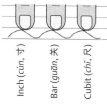

Floating level
Middle level
Deep level

Inch (*cùn*, 寸)   Bar (*guān*, 关)   Cubit (*chǐ*, 尺)   Inch (*cùn*, 寸)   Bar (*guān*, 关)   Cubit (*chǐ*, 尺)

The sunken pulse indicates an interior pattern. A sunken, forceful pulse points to interior repletion; a sunken, forceless pulse points to interior vacuity.

The slow pulse indicates a cold pattern. A slow, forceful pulse indicates cold repletion (note: or repletion heat); a slow, forceless pulse indicates vacuity cold.

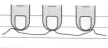

A faint, weak, and rough pulse manifestation in men indicates infertility.

Patients with frequent seminal emission due to excessive exhaustion of seminal fluid usually present with lower abdominal pain, a cold sensation in the penis, painful eye sockets, hair loss, and an extremely vacuous and weak pulse. If the pulse is also scallion-stalk and slow, this indicates seminal loss, blood collapse, or clear-food diarrhea.

A scallion-stalk, stirred, faint, and tight pulse manifestation indicates dual vacuity of yin *and* yang.

If there is a presence of a scallion-stalk, stirred, faint, and tight pulse manifestation, this indicates dual vacuity of *yin* and *yang*; in men, there will be a tendency for seminal emission, and in women, a tendency to dream of having sexual intercourse. Use Cinnamon Twig Decoction Plus Dragon Bone and Oyster Shell (*Guī Zhī Jiā Lóng Gǔ Mǔ Lì Tāng*, 桂枝加龍骨牡蠣湯) to treat this condition.

Drumskin pulse:
Vacuity taxation from essence and blood depletion.

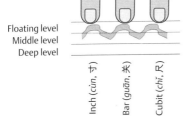

Floating level
Middle level
Deep level

Inch (*cùn*, 寸)   Bar (*guān*, 关)   Cubit (*chǐ*, 尺)

The drumskin pulse indicates blood collapse or seminal loss.

A sunken, small, and slow pulse indicates spleen and kidney debilitation.

If the pulse manifestation is sunken, small, and slow, this indicates spleen and kidney debilitation, and is called deserting *qi*. Patients suffering from deserting *qi* will experience panting while walking, cold hands and feet, abdominal distention and fullness, thin sloppy stools, and indigestion.

A stringlike and large pulse manifestation indicates vacuity taxation from essence and blood depletion.

If the pulse is stringlike and large, this is the pulse manifestation of vacuity taxation from essence and blood depletion. Although the pulse is stringlike, its strength is reduced under heavy pressure. Although the pulse is large, it is hollow; this reduction in strength upon heavy pressure indicates cold. A large but hollow pulse indicates vacuity, which is vacuity and cold contending with each other and binding together; this type of pulse is called a drumskin pulse. The presence of a drumskin pulse in women reveals a tendency for late miscarriage or incessant spotting of menstrual blood. In men, a drumskin pulse reveals blood loss or seminal loss.

■ Chapter 7: Discussion of the Pulse and Signs of Wasting Thirst and Strangury

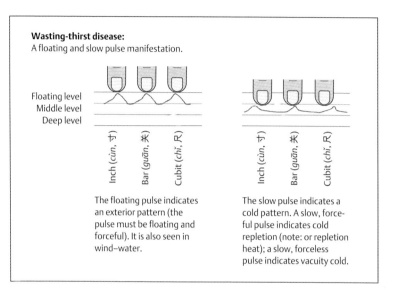

Wasting-thirst disease:
A floating and slow pulse manifestation.

Floating level
Middle level
Deep level

Inch (cùn, 寸)   Bar (guān, 关)   Cubit (chǐ, 尺)

Inch (cùn, 寸)   Bar (guān, 关)   Cubit (chǐ, 尺)

The floating pulse indicates an exterior pattern (the pulse must be floating and forceful). It is also seen in wind–water.

The slow pulse indicates a cold pattern. A slow, forceful pulse indicates cold repletion (note: or repletion heat); a slow, forceless pulse indicates vacuity cold.

Key points emphasized

– Discusses the pulse, signs, and treatment of wasting-thirst and strangury (*lín zhèng*, 淋證).

> *Reverting* yin *disease patients may exhibit wasting-thirst syndrome, which is characterized by thirst that is not relieved by drinking, an upsurge of* qi *into the heart, heart pain, hunger with no desire to eat, and immediate vomiting after eating. If this condition is mistreated with draining precipitation, it will result in incessant diarrhea.*

As for the floating and slow pulse manifestation, the floating quality stands for *yang* vacuity causing *qi* to float upward, and insufficiency of defense *qi*, while the slow quality reveals emptiness of the blood vessels and depletion of construction and *yin*. Dual vacuity of construction and defense and the internal generation of dryness–heat results in the formation of wasting-thirst disease.

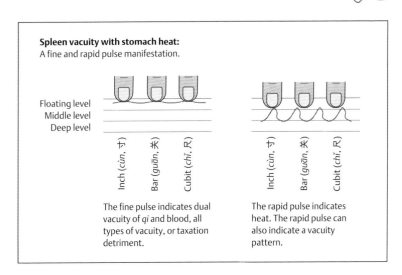

Spleen vacuity with stomach heat:
A fine and rapid pulse manifestation.

Floating level
Middle level
Deep level

Inch (cùn, 寸)
Bar (guān, 关)
Cubit (chǐ, 尺)

Inch (cùn, 寸)
Bar (guān, 关)
Cubit (chǐ, 尺)

The fine pulse indicates dual vacuity of *qi* and blood, all types of vacuity, or taxation detriment.

The rapid pulse indicates heat. The rapid pulse can also indicate a vacuity pattern.

If the instep *yang* pulse is floating and rapid, the floating quality indicates superabundance of stomach *qi*, whereas the rapid speed indicates hyperactivity of stomach heat. Hyperactive stomach heat gives rise to a large food intake with rapid hungering; superabundance of stomach *qi* is fire, which forces water to seep into the urinary bladder, resulting in frequent urination. Stomach heat and stomach *qi* contend with each other and bind together, thereby producing the signs and symptoms of wasting-thirst, which include a large intake of food and drink, and urinary frequency.

> *Fire forces water to seep into the urinary bladder, resulting in frequent urination.*

Men suffering from wasting-thirst disease have thirst with a liking for fluids. Because of kidney *yang* vacuity detriment, the body fluids cannot be steamed, and therefore water cannot be properly transformed. This will result in the production of urine equal to the amount of water consumed. Use Kidney *Qi* Pill (*Shèn Qì Wán*, 腎氣丸) to treat this.

Evil heat gathering and binding in the lower burner will manifest as bloody urine, urinary strangury, and blockage. Intense heat in the urinary bladder can develop into stone strangury disease, which is also commonly known as urinary tract stones. Urine is decocted by this intense heat and forms sandy stones the size of millet grains, obstructing the urinary tract and causing difficult voidings of rough, stagnant urine, and lower abdominal hypertonicity with pain that radiates to the umbilicus.

As for the fine and rapid pulse manifestation, the rapid speed indicates heat, and the fine quality indicates cold. This is caused by vomiting that results in spleen vacuity with stomach heat.

As for the floating and slow instep *yang* pulse, the floating quality indicates *yang* vacuity causing *qi* to float upward, and insufficiency of defense *qi*; the slow speed reveals emptiness of the blood vessels and depletion of construction and *yin*. Dual vacuity of construction and defense and the internal generation of dryness–heat results in the formation of wasting-thirst disease.

If the lesser yin *pulse is rapid, this indicates kidney* yin *vacuity with evil heat intrusion in the lower burner.*

If the lesser *yin* pulse is rapid, this indicates kidney *yin* vacuity with evil heat intrusion in the lower burner; there will also be a tendency for genital sores in women and a tendency for inhibited and painful voidings of rough stagnant urine (*qi* strangury disease) in men.

Strangury disease patients should not be treated with diaphoresis.

As strangury disease is commonly caused by kidney *yin* vacuity detriment and intense heat in the urinary bladder, strangury disease patients should not be treated with diaphoresis. Strong diaphoresis would further consume *yin* and blood, and give rise to bloody urine.

■ Chapter 9: Discussion of the Pulse and Signs of Jaundice, Cold and Heat, and Malaria

Key points emphasized

– Discusses the pulse, signs, and treatment of jaundice, malaria, and mother-of-malaria (*nüè mǔ*, 瘧母).

– If jaundice patients exhibit no pulse manifestation and a cold sensation in the lips and nose, these are signs of heart and spleen *qi* expiry, a condition that is difficult to treat.

– A sunken pulse, thirst with a desire to drink water, and inhibited urination are signs of damp–heat brewing and binding in the center burner, which leads to yellowing. Abdominal distention and fullness, somber yellowing of the body, and vexation and agitation with insomnia are symptoms of jaundice.

– In patients suffering from jaundice, the cause of disease is damp–heat if there is fever, vexation and agitation, panting, and fullness and oppression of the chest and rib-side. If mistreated with the fire-attacking method to induce diaphoresis, instead of resulting in exterior resolution, more heat will be added to the pre-existing heat; the two combined heats will strengthen the fever. However, jaundice is caused by dampness evil, and generalized fever and yellowing (especially fever in the abdomen) is an indication of interior heat. It should be treated with draining precipitation.

– Jaundice should have a treatment course of 18 days. By the 10th day of treatment, the disease condition should show improvement; if, conversely, the disease condition has worsened, it has become very difficult to treat.

– Jaundice accompanied by thirst is damp–heat transforming into dryness, and is an indication of disease evil entering the interior; it is, therefore, hard to treat. A lack of thirst indicates that the disease evil has not yet entered the deeper aspects of the body, which means that the heat is not exuberant, and the condition can thus be treated. If the disease evil is lodged in the construction, blood, or *yin* aspects, there will be vomiting. If the disease evil is lodged in the defense, *qi*, or *yang* aspects, it will manifest as shivering and fever.

– Jaundice should be treated primarily by freeing the urine. If the pulse is floating, this indicates that the disease evil is still in the fleshy exterior, and should be treated with diaphoresis by administering Cinnamon Twig Decoction Plus Astragalus Decoction (*Guì Zhī Jiā Huáng Qí Tāng*, 桂枝加黃耆湯).

– If generalized yellowing of the body occurs in men, and is accompanied by uninhibited urination, this type of yellowing is not caused by damp–heat, but by vacuity taxation due to dual vacuity of *yin* and *yang* instead. One should treat this with Minor Center-Fortifying Decoction (*Xiǎo Jiàn Zhōng Tāng*, 小建中湯).

– Jaundice with abdominal distention and fullness, inhibited urination of a reddish-yellow color, and spontaneous sweating indicates a repletion pattern in which the exterior has already been resolved, but the interior heat is still intense. This condition should be treated with draining precipitation method, by administering Rhubarb, Phellodendron, Gardenia, and Mirabilitum Decoction (*Dà Huáng Huáng Bǎi Zhī Zǐ Máng Xiāo Tāng*, 大黃黃柏栀子芒硝湯).

– Jaundice with uninhibited urination of normal color, abdominal distention and fullness, panting, and shortness of breath indicates vacuity cold in the center burner, and is caused by internal cold–damp. It cannot be mistreated as repletion heat by clearing heat, or else this will result in damage to center *yang* and produce hiccoughs. If hiccoughs arise, they should be treated with Minor Pinellia Decoction (*Xiǎo Bàn Xià Tāng*, 小半夏湯).

In patients suffering from liquor jaundice (*jiǔ dǎn*, 酒疸), the cause of disease is fondness of liquor, which leads to damp–heat brewing internally, and gives rise to inhibited urination, vexation, oppression and restlessness in the heart, heat effusion in the soles, counterflow ascent of stomach *qi* with an inability to eat or drink, and frequent nausea with the desire to vomit. This is known as liquor jaundice.

Some patients suffering from liquor jaundice do not present with fever, but exhibit a quiet and peaceful spirit-affect, absence of deranged speech, abdominal distention and fullness, a desire to vomit, and dryness of the nasal cavity. In those with a floating pulse manifestation, the disease is in the upper portion of the body, and can be treated with emesis. In those with a sunken pulse manifestation, the disease is in the lower portion of the body, and can be treated with precipitation.

> *In those with a floating pulse manifestation, the disease is in the upper portion of the body, and can be treated with emesis. In those with a sunken pulse manifestation, the disease is in the lower portion of the body, and can be treated with precipitation.*

Vexing heat in the heart and a desire to vomit in patients with liquor jaundice reveals that there is a counterflow ascent of disease evil, and should be treated with emesis to rid of the evil.

In patients with liquor jaundice, there is yellowing of the skin of the whole body and glomus obstruction below the heart.

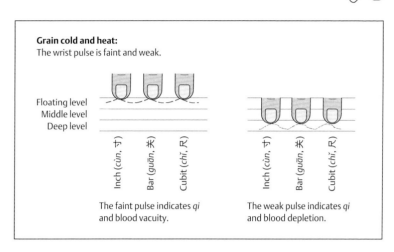

Grain cold and heat:
The wrist pulse is faint and weak.

Floating level
Middle level
Deep level

Inch (cùn, 寸)   Bar (guān, 关)   Cubit (chǐ, 尺)

Inch (cùn, 寸)   Bar (guān, 关)   Cubit (chǐ, 尺)

The faint pulse indicates *qi* and blood vacuity.

The weak pulse indicates *qi* and blood depletion.

If liquor jaundice is treated with draining precipitation, it can turn into black jaundice (*hēi dǎn*, 黑疸), which is characterized by a dark facial complexion, green-blue eyes, scorching heat in the heart, a facial expression likened to having just eaten pickled garlic, black stools (like the color of tar), numbness of the skin, and a floating and weak pulse. Although the eyes are dark, they still contain a yellow color. This condition of black jaundice is caused by the erroneous application of precipitation.

> *If a patient suffering from grain cold and heat presents with a faint and weak pulse, the faint quality indicates* yang qi *vacuity, while the weak quality indicates blood vacuity.*

As for the wrist pulse that is faint and weak, the faint quality indicates a debilitation of *yang qi*, which is characterized by aversion to cold, and the weak quality indicates blood vacuity, which is characterized by fever. If there is absence of fever when there should be fever, there will be aching sinews and bones. If there is an absence of vexation and agitation when there should be vexation and agitation, there will be great sweating (*dà hàn chū*, 大汗出). If the instep *yang* pulse is moderate and slow, this indicates spleen *qi* vacuity with strong stomach *qi*.

> *This is due not to strong stomach* qi, *but to evil heat digesting food.*

If the lesser *yin* pulse is faint, this indicates damaged essence, insufficiency of essence and blood, and kidney *yang* debilitation (which leads to internal exuberance of *yin* cold). Although the patient's spleen and stomach is vacuous, the patient unexpectedly has a good appetite, and also experiences fever with vexation, oppression, distention, and fullness in the abdomen after meals. This is due not to strong stomach *qi*, but to evil heat digesting food; hence, during the onset of disease, the patient will experience a sensation of extreme hunger, and fever and abdominal fullness after meals. Because of damage to the kidney essence and spleen *yang*, the more one eats, the thinner one becomes; this is known as grain cold and heat (*gǔ hán rè*, 穀寒熱).

> *Grain jaundice patients may exhibit a slow pulse, an inability to eat to their fill, or vexation and oppression after eating to their fill.*

Patients with *yang* brightness disease (*yáng míng bìng*, 陽明病) may exhibit a slow pulse, an inability to eat their fill, or vexation and oppression after eating to their fill. If there is dizziness, there will also be inhibited urination; this type of disease is called grain jaundice (*gǔ dǎn*, 穀疸). If abdominal distention shows no improvement after the application of draining precipitation, this is due to spleen and stomach vacuity cold causing an inability to move and transform the essence of grain and water.

> *If the wrist pulse is floating and moderate, the floating quality indicates wind evil, whereas the moderate quality indicates an impediment pattern. Impediment pattern is not wind strike, but rather damp-heat brewing internally in the spleen and causing restlessness of the four limbs. Long-term brewing of damp-heat will turn into jaundice, as damp-heat spilling into the fleshy exterior causes yellowing.*

If the instep *yang* pulse is tight and rapid, the rapid speed denotes heat (intense stomach heat leading to swift digestion with rapid hungering), and the tight quality signifies cold (exuberant cold leading to spleen damage, causing abdominal distention and fullness after meals). A floating pulse in the cubit (*chǐ*) position indicates kidney damage; a tight instep *yang* pulse indicates spleen damage. Wind evil and cold evil contending with each other and binding together causes an upsurge of evil *qi* after meals, which results in dizziness. When food is not moved and transformed, there is glomus obstruction in the stomach, and the turbid *qi* in the stomach will congest and gather in the lower burner, giving rise to inhibited urination, damp-heat pouring downward into the urinary bladder, and damp-heat spilling into the skin and flesh (resulting in yellowing of the whole body). This is known as grain jaundice.

> *Sexual taxation jaundice is caused by sexual taxation damaging the kidney and vacuity taxation.*

If the patient has darkening of the forehead with slight sweating, heat in the palms and soles, an onset of disease at nightfall, urinary urgency, and uninhibited urination, this is caused by sexual taxation damaging the kidney and vacuity taxation, and not by damp-heat. This condition is known as sexual taxation jaundice. In severe cases, there is abdominal swelling (as if filled with water) and distention, which reveals spleen and kidney debilitation, in which case the disease is labeled "untreatable."

If a jaundice patient presents with fever at nightfall, the cause of disease is damp-heat brewing internally. If the patient has no fever in the evening but instead an aversion to cold, he or she is suffering from sexual taxation jaundice. This disease is characterized by urinary urgency, lower abdominal distention and fullness, yellowing of the whole body, darkening of the forehead, and heat in the soles; if one does not recover from this, it will, over a long period of time, turn into black jaundice. Abdominal swelling (as if filled with water) and distention, and black stools with frequent thin sloppy diarrhea are a result of sexual taxation and not of water swelling (*shuǐ zhǒng*, 水腫). For patients with abdominal distention and fullness that is rather difficult to cure, Niter and Alum Powder (*Xiāo Shí Fán Shí Sǎn*, 硝石礬石散) can be used to treat this condition.

In malaria, the pulse manifestation is usually stringlike. If it is stringlike and rapid, this indicates that the evil heat is strong. If the pulse is stringlike and slow, this indicates exuberant cold evil.

The presence of a stringlike, faint, and tight pulse indicates interior food stagnation, which can be treated with draining precipitation. If there is a stringlike and slow pulse manifestation, the warming method should be employed as treatment. A tight and rapid pulse manifestation reveals externally contracted wind–cold, which can be treated with diaphoresis, acupuncture, and moxibustion. If there is a floating and large pulse, emesis can be administered. A pulse that manifests as stringlike and rapid indicates extreme heat engendering wind, which should be treated by consuming sweet and cold food and beverages.

If malaria remains uncured over a long period of time, malarial evil will bind and gather under the rib-side with static blood and phlegm turbidity to form concretions and conglomerations (*zhēng jiǎ*, 癥瘕), goiters, and tumors of the neck. This condition is known as mother-of-malaria, and should be treated with Turtle Shell Decocted Pill (*Biē Jiǎ Jiān Wán*, 鱉甲煎丸).

Malaria accompanied by fever is called warm malaria, which is characterized by a balanced pulse, fever, an absence of aversion to cold, painful and irritable joints, frequent retching, and fever in the morning that is relieved by nightfall. Warm malaria should be treated with White Tiger Decoction Plus Cinnamon Twig Decoction (*Bái Hǔ Jiā Guì Zhī Tāng*, 白虎加桂枝湯).

Malaria accompanied by aversion to cold is usually caused by exuberance of *yin* due to *yang* vacuity, which results in malarial evil stagnating in the *yin* aspect. This condition is known as male malaria (*mǔ nüè*, 牡瘧), and should be treated with Dichroa Leaf Powder (*Shǔ Qī Sǎn*, 蜀漆散).

Various pulse manifestations of malaria

– A stringlike and rapid pulse signifies strong evil heat.

– A stringlike and slow pulse denotes exuberant cold evil.

– A faint and tight pulse manifestation reveals interior food stagnation, which can be treated with draining precipitation.

– In the case of a stringlike and slow pulse, the condition should be treated with the warming method.

– A tight and rapid pulse suggests externally contracted wind–cold, which can be treated with diaphoresis, acupuncture, and moxibustion.

– In the case of a floating and large pulse, the condition can be treated with emesis.

– A stringlike and rapid pulse indicates extreme heat engendering wind, in which case the condition should be treated by consuming sweet and cold food and beverages.

Floating level
Middle level
Deep level

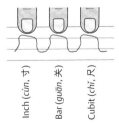

Inch (*cùn*, 寸) Bar (*guān*, 关) Cubit (*chǐ*, 尺)

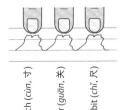

Inch (*cùn*, 寸) Bar (*guān*, 关) Cubit (*chǐ*, 尺)

The stringlike pulse indicates liver and gallbladder disease, phlegm-rheum, all types of pain, or malaria. The stringlike pulse can also signify vacuity.

The tight pulse indicates cold, pain, or abiding food.

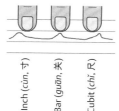

Floating level
Middle level
Deep level

Inch (cùn, 寸) Bar (guān, 关) Cubit (chǐ, 尺)

The slow pulse indicates a cold pattern. A slow, forceful pulse indicates cold repletion (note: or repletion heat); a slow, forceless pulse indicates vacuity cold.

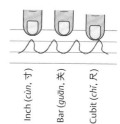

Inch (cùn, 寸) Bar (guān, 关) Cubit (chǐ, 尺)

The rapid pulse indicates heat. The rapid pulse can also indicate a vacuity pattern.

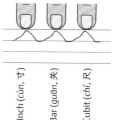

Floating level
Middle level
Deep level

Inch (cùn, 寸) Bar (guān, 关) Cubit (chǐ, 尺)

The floating pulse indicates an exterior pattern (the pulse must be floating and forceful). It is also seen in wind–water.

Chapter 10: Discussion of the Pulse and Signs of Chest Impediment, Heart Pain, Shortness of Breath, and Running Piglet

Key points emphasized

– Discusses the pulse, signs, and treatment of chest impediment, heart pain, shortness of breath, and running piglet disease.

> *During the diagnosis, one should pay attention to the excesses and insufficiencies in the pulse manifestation. If there is a faint (*yang*) and stringlike (*yin*) pulse, this is yang qi insufficiency in the upper burner with yin cold exuberance in the lower burner, which causes yang qi impediment and blockage in the chest, resulting in the condition known as chest impediment.*

Patients with chest impediment experience panting and shortness of breath, cough, chest and back pain, and a sunken and slow pulse that is slightly tight and rapid in the bar (*guān*) position. This is a result of devitalized chest *yang*, retention of rheum in the center burner, and *yin* cold overwhelming the chest. Administer Trichosanthes, Chinese Chive, and White Liquor Decoction (*Guā Lóu Xiè Bái Bái Jiǔ Tāng*, 栝蔞薤白白酒湯) to treat this condition.

Before the onset of chest impediment, the patient appears to be of normal health. When the disease flares up, there is chest pain and shortness of breath. These symptoms are caused by *yin* cold obstructing and stagnating in the chest, and are attributable to repletion.

Running piglet patients experience subjective sensations of *qi* surging straight up from the lower abdomen to the throat. When the disease flares up, there is pain so severe that the patient wants to die; when the disease is no longer active, the patient recovers from the pain and returns to normal. These symptoms are caused by stimulation from fear and fright.

The onset of running piglet disease is characterized by the upsurge of *qi* counterflow, pain in the chest and abdomen, and alternating fever and chills. Use Running Piglet Decoction (*Bēn Tún Tāng*, 奔豚湯) to treat this condition.

> *Among the various disease patterns, there are running piglet, vomiting of pus and blood, fright and terror, and fire evil. These four kinds of diseases are all caused by stimulation from fear and fright.*

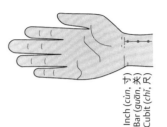

A sunken and slow pulse that is slightly tight and rapid in the bar (*guān*) position.

Floating level
Middle level
Deep level

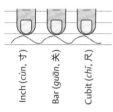

The sunken pulse indicates an interior pattern.
A sunken, forceful pulse points to interior repletion; a sunken, forceless pulse points to interior vacuity.

The slow pulse indicates a cold pattern. A slow, forceful pulse indicates cold repletion (note: or repletion heat); a slow, forceless pulse indicates vacuity cold.

Floating level
Middle level
Deep level

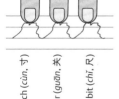

The tight pulse indicates cold, pain, or abiding food.

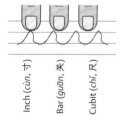

The rapid pulse indicates heat. The rapid pulse can also indicate a vacuity pattern.

■ Chapter 11: Discussion of the Pulse and Signs of Abdominal Fullness, Cold Mounting, and Abiding Food

Key points emphasized

– Discusses the pulse, signs, abdominal fullness, cold mounting (*hán shàn*, 寒疝), and abiding food (*sù shí*, 宿食).
– If the instep *yang* pulse is stringlike, there should be distention and fullness of the stomach duct and abdomen. If the stomach and abdomen are not distended and full, there will be difficult defecation and pain in the rib-side region. The cause of this condition is ascension of vacuity cold counterflow from the lower body to the upper body, and it should be treated with warming medicinals.

If there is no pain upon palpation in patients with abdominal distention and fullness, the condition is attributed to vacuity. If there is pain upon palpation, the condition is attributed to repletion, and can be treated with draining precipitation. If the tongue fur is yellow, this signifies heat in the interior. Using draining precipitation to drain the heat will cause the yellow tongue fur to fade.

Patients with abdominal distention and fullness will experience occasional alleviations and flare-ups of symptoms. This is due to spleen and stomach vacuity cold, and should be treated with warming medicinals.

If the instep *yang* pulse manifestation is tight and floating, the tight quality indicates cold evil and pain, whereas the floating quality signifies vacuity, namely spleen *yang qi* vacuity giving rise to rumbling intestines. The tight quality can also indicate hardness, distention, and fullness of the abdominal region.

> *A pulse that is stringlike and slow in both hands reveals hardness below the heart. If the pulse manifestation is large and tight, this indicates* yin *within* yang, *or vacuity–repletion complex.*

In patients with abdominal distention and fullness, a pulse that is stringlike and slow in both hands reveals hardness below the heart. If the pulse manifestation is large and tight, this indicates *yin* within *yang*, or vacuity–repletion complex, which can be treated with draining precipitation. Abdominal distention and fullness accompanied by pain signifies interior repletion, and should be treated with draining precipitation.

Abdominal distention and fullness that shows no improvement or only slight relief but no real improvement indicates that interior repletion evil has not yet been expelled. One should treat this condition with draining precipitation.

After 10 days of fever in patients with abdominal fullness, the pulse manifestation becomes floating and rapid, and there is a normal intake of food and drink. This means that the disease evil has already entered the interior, and there is concurrent greater *yang* and *yang* brightness disease. One should use Official Magnolia Bark Three Agents Decoction (*Hòu Pò Sān Wù Tāng*, 厚朴三物湯) to drain the evil heat from the stomach and intestines. For severe distention, fullness, and pain of the abdomen, Official Magnolia Bark Seven Agents Decoc-

---

Abdominal distention and fullness

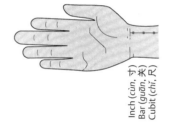

A slow and moderate pulse manifestation can suggest gripping pain in the abdomen.

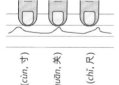

Floating level
Middle level
Deep level

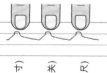

The slow pulse indicates a cold pattern. A slow, forceful pulse indicates cold repletion (note: or repletion heat); a slow, forceless pulse indicates vacuity cold.

The moderate pulse indicates dampness or spleen vacuity.

tion (*Hòu Pò Qī Wù Tāng*, 厚朴七物湯) should be administered to resolve both the exterior and the interior.

> *Patients with abdominal fullness that present with a slow and moderate pulse manifestation will develop gripping pain in the abdomen.*

In patients with abdominal fullness that present with a slow and moderate pulse manifestation, the slowness indicates *yin* cold, whereas the moderate quality indicates *qi* stagnation. Cold evil and *qi* stagnation contending with each other and binding together will lead to gripping pain in the abdomen.

If the pulse manifests as slow and rough, the slowness signifies *yin* cold, while the rough quality indicates insufficiency of construction–blood.

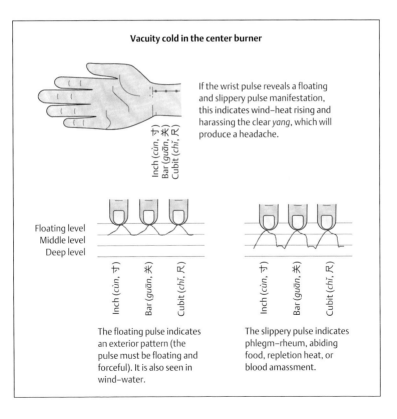

Vacuity cold in the center burner

Inch (*cùn*, 寸)
Bar (*guān*, 关)
Cubit (*chǐ*, 尺)

If the wrist pulse reveals a floating and slippery pulse manifestation, this indicates wind–heat rising and harassing the clear *yang*, which will produce a headache.

Floating level
Middle level
Deep level

Inch (*cùn*, 寸)
Bar (*guān*, 关)
Cubit (*chǐ*, 尺)

Inch (*cùn*, 寸)
Bar (*guān*, 关)
Cubit (*chǐ*, 尺)

The floating pulse indicates an exterior pattern (the pulse must be floating and forceful). It is also seen in wind–water.

The slippery pulse indicates phlegm–rheum, abiding food, repletion heat, or blood amassment.

Patients with vacuity cold in the center burner have the urge to yawn in a subconscious attempt to restore the smooth flow of *yang qi*. If it is accompanied by a runny nose with clear snivel, fever, and a normal facial complexion, this indicates a newly contracted external evil, and sneezing can easily arise.

In patients with vacuity cold in the center burner, since center *yang* is depleted, *yang qi* lacks the force to thrust itself outward. As a result, although there is the urge to sneeze, the patient is unable to do so.

Periumbilical pain in thin and weak patients is caused by wind–cold contraction, which leads to impairment of the spleen and stomach, and results in blocked and bound stools. This condition is attributed to cold bind (hán jié, 寒結). If the condition is mistreated with bitter and cold medicinals to induce offensive precipitation, the center *yang* will be further damaged, causing the upsurge of stomach *qi*. If *qi* does not surge up, it will stay lodged in the center burner and give rise to glomus and fullness below the heart.

At this time, if the patient with vacuity cold in the center burner presents with a stringlike pulse manifestation, it would be accompanied by hypertonicity and pain under the rib-side and a severe aversion to cold.

If the wrist pulse reveals a floating and slippery pulse manifestation, this indicates wind–heat rising and harassing the clear *yang*, which will produce a headache.

If the instep *yang* pulse is moderate and slow, the moderate quality indicates vacuity cold, while the slowness denotes *qi* vacuity. Vacuity and cold contend with each other and bind together in the center burner, giving the patient a desire to eat hot food. If the patient consumes raw and cold food and beverages, the *qi* dynamic will be obstructed, and a sore throat will arise.

If there is a faint pulse that is tight and rough at the middle level of the cubit (*chǐ*) position, the tight quality indicates cold, the faint quality indicates *qi* vacuity, and the rough quality signifies blood vacuity. The presence of this kind of pulse manifestation reveals erroneous treatment involving the use of draining precipitation after the administration of diaphoresis. If the instep *yang* pulse is tight, this is cold in the center burner, which should be treated with the warming method; why would one resort to using diaphoresis and draining precipitation to treat this condition?

> If the pulse manifests as rapid and stringlike, one should administer warm precipitation to dispel the cold.

If the pulse manifestation is floating and tight, it resembles a stringlike pulse in that it feels like a bowstring that has been stretched tight and will not yield when

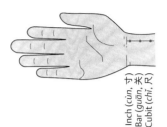

Vacuity cold in the center burner

A faint wrist pulse

Inch (cùn, 寸)
Bar (guān, 关)
Cubit (chǐ, 尺)

A pulse manifestation that is tight and rough in the middle level of the cubit (*chǐ*) position.

This is a result of erroneous treatment involving the use of draining precipitation after the administration of diaphoresis.

heavy pressure is applied. If the pulse manifests as rapid and stringlike, one should administer warm precipitation to dispel the cold. A condition that is characterized by pain under the left or right rib-side and a tight, stringlike pulse is attributed to cold repletion binding and gathering in the center burner, and should be treated with warming medicinals to induce offensive precipitation, such as the administration of Rhubarb and Aconite Decoction (*Dà Huáng Fù Zǐ Tāng*, 大黄附子汤).

> The combination of stringlike and tight pulse qualities indicates the formation of cold mounting (hán shàn, 寒疝).

If the wrist pulse manifests as stringlike and tight, the stringlike quality is caused by external evil obstructing the defensive *yang* and giving rise to stagnation of the defense *qi*, while the tight quality indicates cold and center *yang* vacuity resulting in a lack of appetite. The combination of stringlike and tight pulse qualities indicates the formation of cold mounting (*hán shàn*, 寒疝).

If the instep *yang* pulse manifestation is floating and slow, the floating quality indicates wind and vacuity, while the slowness indicates cold mounting. Cold *qi* binding internally will induce pain in the umbilical region. If, during the onset of cold mounting, there is spontaneous sweating, icy-cold extremities, and a sunken, stringlike pulse, one should use Major Aconite Main Tuber Decoction (*Dà Wū Tóu Tāng*, 大烏頭湯).

> *During the onset of cold mounting, there may be spontaneous sweating, icy-cold extremities, and a sunken, stringlike pulse.*

> **Question:** *If there is an accumulation and stagnation of abiding food in the stomach and intestines, how should it be diagnosed?*
> **Answer:** *If the wrist pulse is floating and large, the application of heavy pressure reveals a rough pulse, and the cubit (chǐ) position is faint and rough, the condition is caused by* qi *stagnation and food accumulation in the stomach and intestines.*
> *A tight wrist pulse that is taut like a twisted rope and unstable in both hands is an indication of abiding food.*

– A tight wrist pulse is an indication of abiding food.

– If the pulse is floating and tight, it indicates a headache induced by externally contracted wind–cold.

– If the pulse is sunken and tight, it indicates indigestion of abiding food in the abdomen.

– If the pulse manifests as slippery and rapid, the pattern is one of interior repletion, and indicates abiding food in the stomach and intestines.

Floating level
Middle level
Deep level

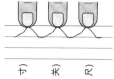

Inch (cùn, 寸)   Bar (guān, 夫)   Cubit (chǐ, 尺)

The floating pulse indicates an exterior pattern (the pulse must be floating and forceful). It is also seen in wind–water.

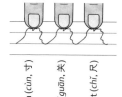

Inch (cùn, 寸)   Bar (guān, 夫)   Cubit (chǐ, 尺)

The tight pulse indicates cold, pain, or abiding food.

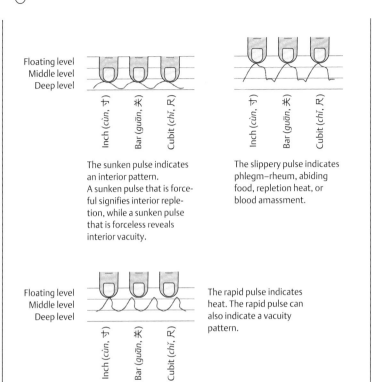

Floating level
Middle level
Deep level

Inch (cùn, 寸)
Bar (guān, 关)
Cubit (chǐ, 尺)

The sunken pulse indicates an interior pattern. A sunken pulse that is forceful signifies interior repletion, while a sunken pulse that is forceless reveals interior vacuity.

Inch (cùn, 寸)
Bar (guān, 关)
Cubit (chǐ, 尺)

The slippery pulse indicates phlegm–rheum, abiding food, repletion heat, or blood amassment.

Floating level
Middle level
Deep level

Inch (cùn, 寸)
Bar (guān, 关)
Cubit (chǐ, 尺)

The rapid pulse indicates heat. The rapid pulse can also indicate a vacuity pattern.

A tight and floating wrist pulse indicates a headache induced by externally contracted wind–cold; a tight and sunken wrist pulse indicates indigestion of abiding food in the abdomen.

If the wrist pulse manifests as slippery and rapid, the pattern is one of interior repletion, and indicates abiding food in the stomach and intestines. The condition should be treated with draining precipitation.

Loss of appetite after a bout of diarrhea is caused by abiding food in the stomach and intestines. It should be treated with draining precipitation.

If, after the application of draining precipitation, there are 6 or 7 days of constipation, unresolved heart vexation, and abdominal distention and pain, this is a result of dry feces adhering to and stagnating in the intestinal tract. The main cause of disease is abiding food.

If there is retention and stagnation of abiding food in the upper portion of the digestive tract, there will be vomiting; this condition should be treated with emesis.

■ Chapter 13: Discussion of the Pulse and Signs of Fright Palpitations, Nosebleed, Blood Ejection, Precipitation of Blood, Chest Fullness, and Static Blood

Key points emphasized

– Discusses the pulse, signs, and treatment of fright palpitations, nosebleeds, blood ejection, precipitation of blood, chest fullness, and static blood.
– If the wrist pulse manifestation is stirred and weak, the stirred quality indicates fright, while the weakness indicates palpitations.
– If the instep *yang* pulse manifests as faint and floating, the floating and forceless quality signifies stomach *qi* vacuity, whereas the faint quality indicates inability to eat. This is the pulse manifestation of fear and dread pattern, which is caused by fright and fear, and characterized by unclear vision and a pulse that pauses temporarily and then resumes.

> **Question:** *If the wrist pulse is tight and the instep* yang *pulse is floating and forceless, this indicates stomach* qi *vacuity. A sunken and tight wrist pulse reveals cold repletion; cold evil congests and gathers in the upper burner and inevitably causes distention and fullness of the chest and belching. In patients with stomach* qi *vacuity, if the instep* yang *pulse manifests as floating and forceless and the lesser* yang *pulse (*shào yáng mài, 少陽脈*) is tight and stringlike, there will be heart palpitations. What is the cause?*
> **Answer:** *This is a result of cold evil and water–damp contending with each other and binding together to cause obstruction in the heart vessels, giving rise to heart palpitations. If pulse diagnosis reveals a rough, soggy, and weak pulse manifestation, this indicates great loss of blood.*

A stringlike and large pulse is the pulse manifestation of vacuity taxation due to essence and blood depletion. Although the pulse is stringlike, its strength is reduced under heavy pressure. The pulse is large, yet empty. A pulse that becomes

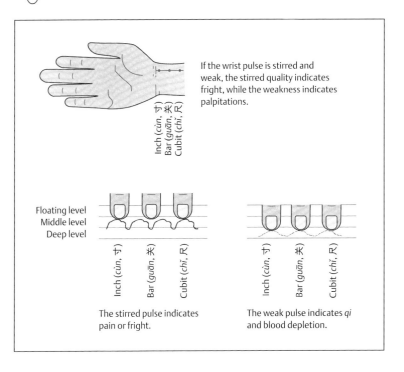

If the wrist pulse is stirred and weak, the stirred quality indicates fright, while the weakness indicates palpitations.

Floating level
Middle level
Deep level

Inch (cùn, 寸) Bar (guān, 关) Cubit (chǐ, 尺)

The stirred pulse indicates pain or fright.

Inch (cùn, 寸) Bar (guān, 关) Cubit (chǐ, 尺)

The weak pulse indicates *qi* and blood depletion.

weak under heavy pressure indicates cold; a large, empty pulse indicates vacuity. This pulse signifies a combination of vacuity and cold, and is known as a drumskin pulse. The presence of a drumskin pulse in women reveals a tendency for late miscarriage or incessant spotting of menstrual blood. In men, a drumskin pulse reveals blood loss.

Patients with blood loss should not be treated with diaphoresis (to resolve the exterior). If the sweating causes severe damage to both *yang qi* and *yin* humor, there will be a fear of cold and shivering of the whole body.

Question: *If there were bleeding from the nose that continued for many days, what would the pulse manifestation be like?*
Answer: *When palpating the pulse, it would feel soft and forceless in the superficial and middle levels, and the cubit (chǐ) position would be floating, large, and forceless. In addition, the eyeballs would be dark yellow in color. These are indications that the bleeding*

has not ceased. When the dark yellow color in the eyeballs has receded and the vision is clear, this means that the bleeding has ceased.

The occurrence of nosebleeds from the spring to the summer season is attributed to greater yang, *while the occurrence of nosebleeds from autumn to winter is attributed to* yang *brightness. This is because in spring and summer,* yang qi *rises and exterior heat is predominant, whereas by autumn and winter,* yang qi *has descended and interior heat is predominant.*

If the inch (cùn) position is faint and weak, and the cubit (chǐ) position is rough, this is attributable to lower body vacuity and upper body repletion.

If the inch (*cùn*) position is faint and weak, and the cubit (*chǐ*) position is rough, the weak quality indicates fever, while the rough quality indicates blood vacuity. The patient will experience cold limbs and mild retching. At this time, there is subjective dizziness without actual dizziness, accompanied by a headache. The pain indicates repletion and is attributable to lower body vacuity and upper body repletion, which gives rise to nosebleeds.

If the greater *yang* pulse (*tài yáng mài*, 太陽脈) manifests as surging, large, and floating, there will inevitably be nosebleeds and blood ejection.

A floating and weak pulse that disappears under heavy pressure reveals vacuous *yang* floating outward.

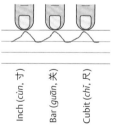

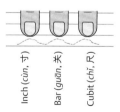

Floating level
Middle level
Deep level

Inch (*cùn*, 寸) Bar (*guān*, 关) Cubit (*chǐ*, 尺)

Inch (*cùn*, 寸) Bar (*guān*, 关) Cubit (*chǐ*, 尺)

The floating pulse indicates an exterior pattern (the pulse must be floating and forceful). It is also seen in wind–water.

The weak pulse indicates *qi* and blood depletion.

If the patient's facial complexion lacks the color of blood, the administration of diaphoresis is prohibited. Sweating will damage the *yin* and consume the blood, giving rise to tension above the forehead, forward-staring eyes that are unable to move, and insomnia.

A floating and weak pulse that disappears under heavy pressure reveals vacuous *yang* floating outward. When *yang* is unable to contain *yin*, there is a downward collapse of blood, resulting in a precipitation of blood. If there is heart vexation accompanied by a dry cough, there will also be blood ejection.

> *If the wrist pulse is faint and weak, this indicates vacuity of both* qi *and blood.*

If the wrist pulse is faint and weak, this indicates vacuity of both *qi* and blood, a tendency for blood ejection in men, and a tendency for precipitation of blood in women. If the above signs are accompanied by vomiting and sweating, this indicates that the condition can still be treated.

If the instep *yang* pulse is faint and weak, and the patient suffers from vomiting and diarrhea in the spring (when stomach *qi* is rising), the condition is also

---

If the patient has a fever accompanied by a faint, small pulse that is on the verge of expiry, this indicates blood ejection, or precipitation of blood and menstrual block in women.

If the patient presents with a slow pulse, this indicates cold–rheum obstruction in the chest.

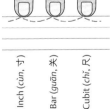

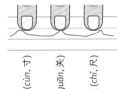

Floating level
Middle level
Deep level

Inch (*cùn*, 寸) Bar (*guān*, 关) Cubit (*chǐ*, 尺)

Inch (*cùn*, 寸) Bar (*guān*, 关) Cubit (*chǐ*, 尺)

The faint pulse indicates *qi* and blood vacuity.

The slow pulse indicates a cold pattern. A slow, forceful pulse indicates cold repletion (note: or repletion heat); a slow, forceless pulse indicates vacuity cold.

relatively easy to treat; if there is *yang* vacuity with water *qi* retention and stagnation, the patient will inevitably have abdominal distention and fullness with inhibited urination.

If the patient presents with fever accompanied by a faint, small pulse that is on the verge of expiry, this indicates blood ejection, or precipitation of blood and menstrual block in women; this condition is a result of cold exuberance from *yang* vacuity. If the patient presents with a slow pulse, this indicates cold rheum obstruction in the chest, which causes frequent belching and ejection of phlegm–drool.

If both the instep *yang* pulse and the lesser *yin* pulse are faint and weak, but the patient does not suffer from vomiting or diarrhea, the condition is caused by blood loss.

A sunken pulse indicates that the disease is in the viscera and bowels and the blood aspect, and that construction–*yin* and defense *qi* are congesting and binding in the interior. If it is accompanied by fullness and oppression in the chest and diaphragm, blood ejection will arise.

A man who is obese but has faint and weak wrist and instep *yang* pulses accompanied by a floating, large, and forceless lesser *yin* pulse will inevitably present with bloody stools and seminal loss. If the above signs are accompanied by urinary pain and distress, there will also be inhibited urination.

If the instep *yang* pulse is stringlike, there will inevitably be bleeding from hemorrhoids.

If the patient exhibits chest distention and fullness, withered lips, a green-blue or purple tongue, a dry mouth and tongue, a desire only to wet the mouth but not to drink, a lack of externally contracted cold or heat, and a pulse that is faint, large, forceless, and slow, and there is no distention and fullness in the abdomen upon palpation but the patient reports abdominal fullness, this is a condition caused by static blood in the interior.

If a condition requires diaphoresis and diaphoresis is not administered, the disease evil will bind and gather in the interior, forming static blood. The patient will experience subjective fever, heart vexation and chest fullness, and a dry mouth with thirst, yet the pulse manifestation will not indicate a heat pattern. This is caused by latent evil heat in the *yin* aspect and internal static blood obstruction. This condition should be treated with draining precipitation.

In the case of precipitation of blood, if there is bleeding followed by defecation, this means that the static blood is not chronic; if defecation occurs first and is then followed by bleeding, this indicates that that the static blood is chronic.

Appendixes

Glossary

Gray highlighting means that the pin yin and Chinese characters for these terms are not included in the running text. As for the non-highlighted terms, the pin yin and Chinese characters are introduced the first time they appear.

PD = *A Practical Dictionary of Chinese Medicine*, Second Edition, Third Printing, 2000: Paradigm Publications, Brookline, Massachusetts, USA.

Abiding food, *sù shí,* 宿食
PD (p. 3): Food and drink accumulating in the stomach and intestines and remaining untransformed for days. It is usually caused by voracious eating or spleen vacuity, and is characterized by abdominal pain and distention, belching of sour fetid *qi*, nausea, aversion to food, constipation or diarrhea, slimy tongue fur, and in some cases, aversion to cold, heat effusion, and headache.

Accumulation, *jī,* 積
PD (p. 3): Gathering; amassment; specifically: (1) a type of abdominal lump; (2) accumulation of food in the digestive tract.

Anterior *yin,* *qián yīn,* 前陰
PD (p. 9): The exterior genitals (male or female). Synonym: "lower *yin*."

***Biān* stone,** *biān shí,* 砭石
An ancient stone acupuncture needle.

Black jaundice, *hēi dǎn,* 黑疸
PD (p. 20): Jaundice characterized by a blackish facial complexion. It arises in persistent jaundice as a result of liver-kidney debilitation and stasis turbidity causing internal obstruction. The body is yellow and lusterless, while the eyes and face

are blackish. There is anguish in the heart, dry skin that is insensitive to scratching, black stool, bladder tension, heat in the underside of the feet, and a weak floating pulse. In severe cases, the abdomen is distended as if containing water, the face is puffy, and pain in the spine prevents the patient from standing erect.

Blood amassment, *xù xuè*, 蓄血
PD (p. 24): A greater *yang* cold damage pattern in which evil heat enters the interior to contend with the blood, causing stasis heat amassing and binding internally and manifesting in the form of smaller-abdominal [lower abdominal] pain and distention, heat effusion and aversion to cold, clear-mindedness in the daytime that gives way to delirious raving, mania, confused speech, and vociferation and violent behavior at night.

Blood chamber, *xuè shì*, 血室
PD (p. 25): 1. The uterus. 2. The thoroughfare (*chong*) vessel. 3. The liver.

Blood collapse, *wáng xuè*, 亡血
PD (p. 26): Acute, critical vacuity of the blood.

Blood ejection, *tù xuè*, 吐血
PD (p. 29): Ejection of blood through the mouth; vomiting or expectoration of blood (i.e., respiratory tract or digestive tract bleeding); sometimes defined as being associated with neither the sound of retching or of coughing.

Body-inches, *cùn*, 寸
PD (p. 41): A proportional unit of measurement used to determine the location of acupuncture points on the body, calculated from the length of specific body parts according to the finger standard and bone standard.

Cinnabar field, *dān tián*, 丹田
PD (p. 62): 1. An area three body-inches below the umbilicus, believed by Daoists to be the chamber of essence (semen) in males and the uterus in females. 2. Any of three mustering positions in *qi-gong*, including the lower cinnabar field located below the umbilicus, the middle cinnabar field located in the pit of the stomach (scrobiculus cordis), and the upper cinnabar field located in the center of the brow.

Clamoring stomach, *cáo zá*, 嘈雜
PD (p. 63): A sensation of emptiness and burning in the stomach duct or heart [region] described as being like hunger but not hunger, and like pain but not

pain, and accompanied by belching, nausea, swallowing of upflowing acid, and fullness.

Clouding reversal, *hūn jué*, 昏厥
PD (p.75): Sudden loss of consciousness and collapse, sometimes accompanied by reversal cold of the limbs. Clouding reversal is usually of short duration as in various reversal patterns; the patient returns to consciousness without hemiplegia or deviation of the eyes and mouth as occurs in wind stroke. In rare cases, it continues, as in death-like reversal. Causes include *qi* vacuity, blood vacuity, phlegm turbidity harassing the upper body, ascendant liver *yang*, summerheat stroke, and tetanic diseases such as child fright wind and epilepsy.

Cold bind, *hán jié*, 寒結
PD (p.77): Constipation arising when spleen-kidney *yang* vacuity causes *yin* cold to congeal and bind, reducing warmth and movement of food. Also known as "cold constipation."

Cold mounting, *hán shàn*, 寒疝
Acute abdominal pain caused by spleen and stomach vacuity cold, postpartum blood vacuity, or contraction of wind-cold evil, which can all cause evil *qi* to enter the interior, and then bind and gather in the stomach duct and abdomen. It is characterized by cold sweating, reversal cold of the four limbs, gripping pain in the abdomen, numbness of the four limbs, and a sunken, tight pulse.

PD (p.82): Accumulation of cold evil in the abdomen arising from repeated wind-cold contractions that in turn stem either from vacuity cold in the spleen and stomach or from postpartum blood vacuity. Characterized by cold in the umbilical region, cold sweating, and counterflow cold in the limbs. The pulse is sunken and tight.

Concretions and conglomerations, *zhēng jiǎ*, 癥瘕
PD (p.92): Two of four kinds of abdominal masses (concretions, conglomerations, accumulations, and gatherings) associated with pain and distention. Concretions and accumulations are masses of definite form and fixed location, associated with pain of fixed location. They stem from disease in the viscera and blood aspect. Conglomerations and gatherings are masses of indefinite form, which gather and dissipate at irregular intervals and are attended by pain of unfixed location; they are attributed to disease in the bowels and *qi* aspect. Concretions and conglomerations chiefly occur in the lower burner, and, in many cases, are the result of gynecological diseases.

Construction-blood, *yíng xuè,* 營血
See "Construction *qi.*"

Construction *qi,* *yíng qì,* 營氣
PD (p.96): Construction 營 *yíng*: An abbreviation for construction *qi,* which is an essential *qi* formed from the essence of food and which flows in the vessels. Construction is considered to be an aspect of blood.

Conveyance, *chuán dǎo,* 傳導
PD (p.340): "Large intestine holds the office of conveyance, whence mutation emanates" (大腸者,傳導之官也,變化出焉): From *Elementary Questions.* The large intestine takes the waste passed on from the small intestine, and conveys it downward to the anus, further transforming it as it does so. Statements such as "large intestine governs transformation and conveyance of waste" and "large intestine governs conveyance" derive from this.

Defense *qi,* wèi qì, 衛氣
PD (p.121): A *qi* described as being "fierce, bold, and uninhibited," unable to be contained by the vessels and therefore flowing outside them. In the chest and abdomen it warms the organs, whereas in the exterior it flows through the skin and flesh, regulates the opening and closing of the interstices, and keeps the skin lustrous and healthy, thereby protecting the fleshy exterior and preventing the invasion of external evils.

Deserting *qi,* tuō qì, 脱氣
PD (p.124): Debilitation of *yang qi* in vacuity taxation disease.

Diaphoresis, *hàn fǎ,* 汗法
PD (p.599): Inducing perspiration as a method of resolving the exterior. It involves the use of acrid dissipating medicinals that promote outthrust and effusion to open and discharge the interstices and expel the evil from the body (skin and body hair), before it enters the interior. One of the eight methods of medicinal treatment.

Draining precipitation, *xiè xià fǎ,* 瀉下法
See "Precipitation."

Dry retching, *gān ǒu,* 乾嘔
PD (p.156): Going through the motions of vomiting without bringing up food, despite possible foaming drool. Attributed to stomach vacuity counterflow *qi* or stomach heat.

Ejection of foamy drool, *tū xián mò,* 吐涎沫

PD (p.170): Copious drooling or vomiting of foamy drool, attributable to rheum evil.

Emesis, *tù fǎ,* 吐法

PD (p.170): Synonym: "ejection." One of the eight methods of medicinal treatment. Refers to induction of vomiting, either by medicinals or by mechanical means (e.g., tickling the throat with a feather) in order to expel collected phlegm or lodged food. This method may also be used to treat poisoning, provided treatment is administered swiftly after ingestion of the toxic substance.

Essence-spirit, *jīng shén,* 精神

PD (p.179): Essence and spirit considered together; the manifestation of the life force. Note: The expression *jīng shén* as colloquially used in Chinese is roughly the equivalent of the English 'energy' (colloquial sense) or 'vitality.' It has also come to be used in modern psychology as the equivalent of the English 'mind.'

Evil block, *xié bì,* 邪閉

During the course of disease progression, due to insufficiency of the right *qi,* the evil *qi* will enter deeper into the body and become harder to expel. The evil *qi* will obstruct the supply and distribution of yin, yang, *qi,* and blood; consequently, this will result in a disease condition where the functions of the bowels and viscera are impaired.

Qi block, cold block, heat block, fire block, *qì bì* (氣閉), *hán bì* (寒閉), *rè bì* (热閉), *huǒ bì* (火閉): When the right *qi* of the body is insufficient, *qi* stagnation, cold evil, heat evil, and/or fire evil can all give rise to block patterns.

Excess among the five minds, *wǔ zhì guò jí,* 五志過極

PD (p.181): A potentially evil excess of one or more of the five minds (basic mental/emotional activities) (joy, anger, anxiety, thought, fear).

Female malaria, *pìn nüè,* 牝瘧

PD (p.197): Malaria in patients with *yang* vacuity with the malarial evil lying in the lesser *yin* channel, characterized by pronounced shivering with little or no heat effusion, pale white complexion, and regular episodes.

Five minds, *wǔ zhì,* 五志

PD (p.205): Joy, anger, anxiety, thought, fear. These are five basic forms of mental and emotional activity, which in excess can cause disease.

Fleshy exterior, *jī biǎo*, 肌表
PD (p.211): The exterior of the body comprised of the skin and flesh and the face, neck, back, abdomen, and limbs.

Flooding, *bēng zhōng*, 崩中
PD (p.211): Heavy menstrual flow or abnormal bleeding via the vagina (uterine bleeding), usually occurring in puberty or at menopause, and attributed to insecurity of the thoroughfare (*chōng*) and controlling (*rèn*) vessels, which may stem from a variety of causes.

Fox-creeper disease, *hú huò bìng*, 狐惑病
A disease pattern primarily caused by damp–heat toxic evil invading the body and giving rise to damp–heat brewing internally. Manifestations include ulcers of the throat region and the anterior and posterior *yin*. Since patients often exhibit spirit-affect (*shén qíng*, 神情) delusions, and fidgetiness when lying down, this illness is thus called fox-creeper disease.

PD (e-book): Roughly equivalent to Behcet's syndrome, which is a group of symptoms of unknown etiology that occur especially in young men and include especially ulcerative lesions of the mouth and genitalia and inflammation of the eye (as uveitis and iridocyclitis)—called also Behcet disease.

Gao-huang, *gāo huāng*, 膏肓
PD (p.239): The region below the heart and above the diaphragm. When a disease is said to have entered the *gao-huang*, it is difficult to cure.

Gathering, *jù*, 聚
PD (p.240): A type of abdominal lump. See "Concretions and conglomerations."

Glomus, *pǐ*, 痞
PD (p.242): A localized, subjective feeling of fullness and blockage.

Grain jaundice, *gǔ dǎn*, 穀疸
PD (e-book): Jaundice due to dietary irregularities.

Great Ravine, *tài xī*, 太谿
KI-3 (name of an acupuncture point on the kidney channel).

Great sweating, *dà hàn*, 大汗
PD (p.248): The flow of sweat in large amounts.

Great sweating, *dà hàn chū*, 大汗出
PD (p. 248): One of the four greatnesses associated with *yang* brightness channel patterns.

Greater *yang* disease, *tài yáng bìng*, 太陽病
One of the six-channel disease patterns. This disease pattern is primarily caused by exposure to wind–cold, which leads to disharmony of construction (*yíng*, 營) and defense (*wèi*, 衛). It can be categorized into exterior repletion and exterior vacuity types. The main symptoms are aversion to cold, headache, stiffness of the nape, and a floating pulse.
   PD (p. 246): Any of a number of diseases affecting greater *yang*.

Greater *yang* pulse, *tài yáng mài*, 太陽脈
See "Three positions and nine indicators."

Green-blue, *qīng*, 青
PD (p. 248): Green, blue, or greenish blue. This color is classically described as "the color of new shoots of grass," but in context of the complexion, for example, it is more often than not a color that would be more naturally described, in English, as blue.

Hard tetany, *gāng jìng*, 剛痙
PD (p. 254): A tetany pattern characterized by heat effusion, absence of sweating, aversion to cold, rigidity of the neck, shaking heat, clenched jaw, and hypertonicity or convulsions of the extremities (in severe cases, arched-back rigidity), and a tight, stringlike pulse.
   PD (p. 607): Distinction is made between soft tetany and hard tetany, the former being distinguished from the latter by the presence of sweating and absence of aversion to cold.

Heart spirit, *xīn shén*, 心神
PD (p. 271): The spirit that is governed by the heart.

Impediment pattern, *bì zhèng*, 痹證
A disease caused by the invasion of the viscera and bowels or of the channels and network vessels by three types of evil *qi* (wind, cold, and dampness). The main symptoms are swelling and distention of the joints or flesh, and pain. Similar to rheumatic arthritis and rheumatoid arthritis.
   PD (p. 294): Blockage of the channels arising when wind, cold, and dampness invade the fleshy exterior and the joints, and manifesting in signs such as joint pain, sinew and bone pain, and heaviness or numbness of the limbs.

Interstices, *còu lǐ*, 腠理
PD (p. 317): An anatomical of unclear identity, explained in modern dictionaries as being the "grain" of the skin, flesh, and organs or the connective tissue in the skin and flesh. *Elementary Questions,* "Clear *yang* effuses through the interstices." Usage of the term suggests that the interstices correspond to the sweat ducts in Western medicine.

Instep *yang* pulse, *fū yáng mài*, 趺陽脈
One of the palpation areas of the Three Positions and Nine Indicators diagnostic method. Its location is on the dorsum of the foot, between the two tendons in front of the ankle joint. It is the arterial pulse located approximately 1.5 body-inches (*cùn*, 寸) in front of Ravine Divide point (*jiě xī*, 解谿).

PD (p. 309): One of the three positions and nine indicators. A pulse 1.5 body-inches in front of ST-41 (*jiě xī*, Ravine Divide) on the upper side of the foot. The instep pulse lies on the foot *yang* brightness (*yáng míng*) stomach channel, and indicates the state of the stomach and spleen.

Jaundice, *huáng dǎn*, 黃疸
The internal brewing of spleen and stomach dampness evil causes stomach and intestinal disharmony, and the outward spilling of bile into the fleshy exterior. The main symptoms are yellowing of the body, eyes, and urine. Clinically, it can be classified into two major types—*yang* jaundice and *yin* jaundice.

PD (p. 322): A condition characterized by the three classic signs of yellow skin, yellow eyes, and yellow urine, i.e., generalized yellowing of the body, yellowing of the whites of the eyes (sclera), and darker-than-normal urine. Jaundice arises when contraction of seasonal evils or dietary irregularities cause damp-heat or cold-damp to obstruct the center burner, and prevents bile from flowing according to its normal course.

Joint-running wind, *lì jié bìng*, 厲節病
Constitutional liver and kidney depletion in conjunction with contraction of external evil leads to disease evil congesting and gathering to form heat, thus giving rise to joint-running wind. It manifests as emaciation, swelling of the feet and lower legs, and joint pain with inability to bend and stretch voluntarily.

PD (p. 322): Synonyms: white tiger joint-running wind; pain wind. A disease described in *Essential Prescriptions of the Golden Coffer* (*Jīn Guì Yào Lüè*, 金匱要略), characterized by redness and swelling of the joints, with acute pain and difficulty bending and stretching. Joint-running wind is attributed to transformation of wind-cold-damp into heat in patients suffering from liver-kidney vacuity, and falls within the scope of impediment.

Lesser abdomen, *shào fù,* 少腹
PD (p. 343): The lateral lower abdomen, i.e., sides of the lower abdomen.

Lesser *yin* pulse, *shào yīn mài,* 少陰脈
One of the palpation areas of the Three Positions and Nine Indicators diagnostic method. It is the arterial pulse 1.5 body-inches above the medial aspect of the ankle joint. It is approximately 1.5 body-inches above Great Ravine (*tài xī* 太谿) *point.*
   PD: See "Three Positions and Nine Indicators."

Lesser *yang* pulse, *shào yáng mài,* 少陽脈
See "Three Positions and Nine Indicators."

Life gate, *mìng mén,* 命門
PD (p. 346): A physiological entity of disputed morphological identity. The term "life gate" first appeared in *The Inner Canon,* where it refers to the eyes. Reference to a "life gate" as an internal organ first appeared in *The Classic of Difficult Issues,* which states, "The two kidneys are not both kidneys. The left one is the kidney, and the right is the life gate." In the Ming and Qing dynasties, various theories were put forward: a) both kidneys contain the life gate; b) the space between the kidneys is the life gate; c) the life gate is the stirring *qi* between the kidneys; d) the life gate is the root of original *qi* and the house of fire and water; e) the life gate is the fire of earlier heaven or the true *yang* of the whole body; f) the life gate is the gate of birth, i.e., the "birth gate" in women and the "essence gate" in men.

Lily disease, *bǎi hé bìng,* 百合病
A disease pattern caused by heart and lung yin vacuity. Clinical manifestations include signs of internal heat, such as taciturnity, a desire to sleep but being unable to sleep, a desire to walk but an inability to walk, a desire to eat but being unable to eat, (subjective sensations of) cold and heat that, an occasionally disquieted spirit-mind (*shén zhì,* 神志), or talking to one's self, accompanied by a bitter taste in the mouth, reddish urine, and a rapid pulse. Similar to neurasthenia, or to the vacuity patterns seen in the sequelae of certain febrile diseases.

Liquid, *jīn,* 津
PD (p. 348): The thinner fluids of the human body.

Liquor jaundice, *jiǔ dǎn,* 酒疸
PD (p. 349): Jaundice arising when excessive liquor consumption gives rise to steaming depressed damp-heat that causes bile leakage. Liquor jaundice is characterized by yellowing of the body and eyes with red macules on the face, anguish, heat, and pain in the heart, dry nose, abdominal fullness with no desire to eat, and periodic desire to vomit.

Lodged rheum, *liú yǐn,* 留飲
PD (p. 366): A form of phlegm-rheum. Persistent rheum evil that fails to transform. Lodged rheum may occur in different parts of the body.

Lower abdomen, *xiǎo fù,* 小腹
PD (p. 541): Synonym: "smaller abdomen." The part of the abdomen below the umbilicus. Compare with "lesser abdomen."

Lower *yin,* *xià yīn,* 下陰
See "Anterior *yin.*"

Lump glomus, *pǐ kuài,* 痞塊
PD (p. 242): Glomus lump: Any palpable abdominal mass. These are classified in ancient literature as concretions, conglomerations, accumulations, and gatherings (*zhēng jiǎ jī jù,* 癥瘕積聚), sometimes being given more specific names as "strings and aggregations" or "deep-lying beam."

Male malaria, *mǔ nüè,* 牡瘧
PD (p. 384): The character 牡 (male) is held to be a mistranscription of 牝 (female). See "Female malaria."

Mother-of-malaria, *nüè mǔ,* 瘧母
PD (p. 399): Lump glomus occurring in enduring malaria; attributed to stubborn phlegm with static blood binding under the rib-side.

Oblique running pulse, *xié fēi mài,* 斜飛脈
PD (p. 418): An anomaly in the position of the wrist pulse in which the pulse runs from the cubit position over the posterior face of the styloid process of the radius toward LI-4 (*hé gǔ,* Union Valley).

Phlegm-drool, *tán xián,* 痰涎
PD (p. 436): Phlegm-rheum, especially thin white, usually copious fluid ejected via the mouth. "Phlegm" refers to thick fluid, whereas "drool" refers to thin fluid.

Phlegm rale, *tán míng*, 痰鳴
PD (p. 440): An abnormal breathing sound produced by the presence of phlegm in the airways.

Physical cold, *xíng hán*, 形寒
PD (p. 444): Outwardly manifest signs of cold, e.g., aversion to cold, desire for warm beverages, curled-up lying posture, cold limbs, etc.

Posterior *yin*, *hòu yīn*, 後陰
PD (p. 447): The anus.

Precipitation, *xià fǎ*, 下法
PD (p. 459): One of the eight methods of medicinal treatment. The stimulation of fecal flow to expel repletion evils and remove accumulation and stagnation.

Precipitation of blood, *xià xuè*, 下血
PD (p. 460): Bloody stool, especially when severe.

Pulse on the back of the wrist, *fǎn guān mài*, 反關脈
PD (p. 473): A congenital anomaly in which the radial pulse is located on the posterior face of the medial styloid process. Also known as "dorsal styloid pulse."

Ravine Divide, *jiě xī*, 解谿
ST-41 (name of an acupoint on the stomach channel).

Reversal cold of the extremities, *shǒu zú jué lěng*, 手足厥冷
PD (p. 505): Synonyms: counterflow cold of the extremities; counterflow cold of the limbs; reversal cold of the limbs; limb reversal. Pronounced cold in the extremities up to the knees and elbows or beyond, as occurs in *yang* collapse or internal heat evil block. Reversal cold of the extremities is similar to lack of warmth in the extremities. However, the latter differs in that it is less pronounced, does not reach as far as the knees and elbows, and is observed in general *yang* vacuity patterns. Reversal cold of the extremities is called *reversal* because *yang qi* recedes away from the extremities. Distinction is made between cold and heat.

Reversal pattern, *jué zhèng*, 厥證
Usually refers to clouding of the heart spirit due to original *qi* vacuity, effulgent liver *yang*, or excessive mental stimulation. The main manifesting symptoms are sudden fainting, loss of consciousness, and reversal cold of the four limbs.

PD (p. 505): Any condition with a) clouding collapse (fainting) and loss of consciousness and/or b) reversal cold of the limbs (marked cold in the extremities).

Reverse-flow, *jué nì*, 厥逆
PD (p. 505): 1. Reversal cold of the extremities. 2. Acute pain in the chest with sudden cold of the lower extremities, heart vexation, inability to eat, and a rough pulse. 3. A kind of enduring headache.

Right *qi*, *zhèng qì*, 正氣
PD (p. 507): 1. True *qi*, especially in opposition to disease. Right *qi* is the active aspect of all components including the organs, blood, fluids, and essence and the above-mentioned forms of *qi* in maintaining health and resisting disease. Right *qi* stands in opposition to evil *qi*, which is any entity in its active aspect of harming the body. 2. The normal *qi* of the seasons, warmth in the spring, heat in summer, coolness in autumn, and cold in winter.

Running piglet, *bēn tún*, 賁豚
The character 賁, pronounced "*bì*," is the same as the character 贲 (*bēn*). A disease caused chiefly by stimulation from fear and fright. The patient will have subjective sensations of *qi* surging straight up from the lower abdomen to the throat, accompanied by pain in the chest and abdomen, and alternating fever and chills. When the disease flares up, there is pain so severe that the patient wants to die; when the disease is no longer active, the patient recovers from the pain and returns to normal.

PD (p. 510): One of the five accumulations (kidney accumulation). A sensation of upsurge from the lower abdomen to the chest and throat, accompanied by gripping abdominal pain, oppression in the chest, rapid breathing, dizziness, heart palpitations, and heart vexation.

Sea of marrow, *suǐ hǎi*, 髓海
PD (p. 517): One of the four seas. The brain.

Shortage of *qi*, *shǎo qì*, 少氣
PD (p. 529): Weak, short, hasty breathing, a weak voice, and a tendency to take deep breaths in order to continue speaking; mainly attributable to visceral *qi* vacuity, especially of center and lung-kidney *qi*, but also observed in phlegm turbidity, water-rheum, food stagnation, and *qi* stagnation.

Six excesses, *liù yín*, 六淫
PD (p.535): Excess or untimeliness of the six *qi* (wind, cold, summerheat, damp, dryness, and fire) that invade the body through the exterior to cause disease. Wind diseases are most common in spring, summerheat in summer, damp disease in long summer, dryness diseases in autumn, and cold diseases in winter.

Skin water, *pí shuǐ*, 皮水
PD (p.536): Water swelling of gradual onset that engulfs the fingers, associated with drum-like enlargement of the abdomen, with absence of both sweating and thirst, and with a floating pulse. Skin water is attributed to spleen vacuity with severe dampness causing water to spill into the skin.

Soft tetany, *róu jìng*, 柔痓
PD (p.544): A tetany pattern characterized by generalized heat [effusion], sweating, rigidity of the neck, shaking of the heat [sic: should be head], clenched jaw, hypertonicity of the extremities, arched-back rigidity, and a slow, sunken pulse.

PD (p.607): Distinction is made between soft tetany and hard tetany, the former being distinguished from the latter by the presence of sweating and absence of aversion to cold.

Sores, *chuāng yáng bìng*, 瘡瘍病
PD (p.545–546): 1. A generic term for diseases of external medicine, such as welling-abscess (*yōng*), flat-abscess (*jū*), clove sore (*dīng chuāng*), boil (*jié*), streaming sore (*liú zhù*), flowing phlegm (*liú tán*), and scrofula (*luǒ lì*), generally caused by toxic evils invading the body, evil heat scorching the blood, and congestion of *qi* and blood. 2. In a wider sense, the term sore includes shallow skin diseases such as scab (*jiè*), lichen (*xiǎn*), and cinnabar toxin (*dān dú*).

Spirit-affect, *shén qíng*, 神情
PD (p.551): The spirit and the outwardly manifest emotions, as seen in the facial expression.

Spirit-mind, *shén zhì*, 神志
PD (p.551): The spirit.

Stomach duct, *wǎn*, 脘 (or *wèi wǎn*, 胃脘)
PD (p.576): Synonym: "venter." The stomach cavity and adjoining sections of the small intestine and gullet. The stomach duct is divided into the upper, center, and lower stomach ducts.

Strangury, *lín*, 淋
PD (p.583): A disease pattern characterized by urinary urgency, frequent short painful rough voidings, and dribbling incontinence. Distinction is made between stone strangury (which also includes sand strangury), *qi* strangury, blood strangury, unctuous strangury, and taxation strangury, known collectively as "the five stranguries."

Sudden death-like reversal, *cù shī jué*, 卒屍厥
Cù, 卒, means "sudden"; *jué*, 厥, means "reversal pattern." *Cù shī jué*, 卒屍厥, means sudden clouding reversal (*hūn jué*, 昏厥).

PD (p.119): Death-like reversal: Clouding reversal and reversal cold in the limbs giving the patient a death-like appearance. Though unconscious, the patient has a pulse.

Sudden turmoil, *huò luàn*, 霍亂
PD (p.61 and 587): Synonym: cholera. A disease characterized by simultaneous vomiting and diarrhea, usually followed by severe cramps. Cholera in Chinese medicine includes what modern Western medicine calls cholera and acute gastroenteritis presenting with the same signs.

Tael, *liǎng*, 兩
PD (p.345): A unit of weight traditionally equal to one sixteenth of a catty (*jīn*, 斤), now equal to 31.25 g.

Taxation damage, *láo shāng*, 勞傷
PD (p.603): 1. Overexertion, intemperate living (including dietary irregularities and sexual intemperance), or the seven affects (emotional imbalance) as a cause of disease. Synonym: "taxation fatigue."

Taxation detriment, *láo sǔn*, 勞損
PD (p.603): Any pattern caused by taxation which in turn causes vacuity detriment to *yin-yang*, *qi*-blood, or the organs. Taxation is the cause, whereas detriment is the resulting pattern. Taxation detriment is also used as a generic name for "vacuity taxation" and "vacuity detriment."

Tetany, *jìng bìng*, 痙病
The main cause of this disease is external evil invading the body. The symptoms are attributed to dryness or wind. Exuberant heat causing damage to *yin* or the misuse of emesis, diaphoresis, and precipitation can all lead to the formation of tetany. The clinical manifestations of tetany are a hot body with cold feet (aver-

sion to cold accompanied by a hot head, a red face, and red eyes), stiffness of the neck and nape, arched-back rigidity, a clenched jaw, and a pulse that is sunken and fine, or racing and rapid.

PD (p.606): Severe spasm such as rigidity in the neck, clenched jaw, convulsions of the limbs, and arched-back rigidity. Repletion patterns are attributed to wind, cold, dampness, phlegm, or fire congesting the channels, whereas vacuity patterns occur when excessive sweating, loss of blood, or constitutional vacuity causes *qi* vacuity, shortage of blood, and insufficiency of the fluids, depriving the sinews of nourishment and allowing internal wind to stir. Distinction is made between soft tetany and hard tetany, the former being distinguished from the latter by the presence of sweating and absence of aversion to cold.

Thermoplegia, *yē*, 暍

Pronounced "*hè*." This is summerheat stroke. Refers to the symptoms of stroke from summerheat evil during the blazing heat of summer. Manifests as generalized fever, profuse sweating (or absence of sweating), sudden loss of consciousness, nausea and vomiting, vexation and agitation, a somber white facial complexion, and a rapid and fine pulse, or coma, convulsion of the limbs, and a clenched jaw.

Thermoplegia is a disease primarily caused by contraction of summerheat–heat. Due to the fumigation and steaming of summerheat–heat, there is profuse sweating and the interstices (*còu lǐ*, 腠理) are loose and empty. As a result, there is aversion to cold and fear of cold. Since summerheat–heat is a fire heat evil, the patient will present with generalized fever. Since summerheat–heat damages the fluids, the patient will present with thirst. In thermoplegia, the pulse will manifest as stringlike and fine, or scallion-stalk and slow. One should use White Tiger Decoction (*Bái Hǔ Tāng*, 白虎湯) to treat this condition.

Three Positions and Nine Indicators, *sān bù jiǔ hòu*, 三部九候

PD (p.610):

1. From *Elementary Questions*: An ancient pulse-taking scheme. The three positions are three areas on the head, upper limbs, and lower limbs, each having three pulse points (indicators), which in most cases can be located by the acupuncture point located at the site. See the list below.

   Head
   – Greater Yang (*tài yáng*)
   – TB-21 (*ěr mén*, Ear Gate)
   – ST-4 (*dì cāng*, Earth Granary)
   – ST-5 (*dà yíng*, Great Reception)

Upper limbs
- wrist pulse
- HT-7 (*shén mén*, Spirit Gate)
- LI-4 (*hé gŭ*, Union Valley)

Lower limbs
- LR-10 (*zú wŭ lĭ*, Foot Five Li) in men and LR-3 (*tài chōng*, Supreme Surge) in women
- SP-11 (*jī mén*, Winnower Gate)
- ST-42 (*chōng yáng*, Surging Yang)
- KI-3 (*tài xī*, Great Ravine)

2. From *The Classic of Difficult Issues*: An ancient pulse-taking scheme. In the context of the wrist pulse, the inch, bar, cubit positions are the three positions, and the superficial level, mid-level, and deep level of each of these are the nine indicators.

Torpid intake, *nà dāi*, 納呆
PD (p.621): Synonym: "torpid stomach." Impairment of the stomach's governing of intake. Torpid intake is attributable to spleen-stomach vacuity or to damp-heat obstruction and is characterized by indigestion and poor appetite, and in some cases, by a sensation of bloating.

Torpid stomach, *wèi dāi*, 胃呆
See "Torpid intake."

Two yin, *èr yīn*, 二陰
PD (p.635): Anus and genitals.

Vacuity detriment, *xū sŭn*, 虛損
PD (p.646): Any form of severe chronic insufficiency of *yin-yang*, *qi*-blood, and bowels and viscera, arising through internal damage by the seven affects, taxation fatigue, diet, excesses of drink and sex, or enduring illness.

Vacuity taxation, *xū láo*, 虛勞
PD (p.651): Any pattern of severe vacuity (of *qi*, blood, or the organs), including notably steaming bone and consumption.

Veiling dizziness, *xuàn mào*, 眩冒
Dizziness with clouding of the head.

Vexing heat in the five centers, *wǔ xīn fán rè*, 五心煩熱

PD (p.655): Vexing heat in the five hearts: Palpable heat in the palms of the hand and soles of the feet, and subjective feeling of heat in the chest. Vexing heat in the five hearts is observed in vacuity detriment and consumption, and arises from effulgent *yin* vacuity fire, vacuity heat failing to clear after illness, or internally depressed fire-heat.

Warm malaria, *wēn nüè*, 溫瘧

PD (p.664): Malaria characterized by generalized heat [effusion], with aversion to cold less pronounced than heat effusion, headache, thirst with taking of fluids, constipation and reddish urine, inhibited sweating, joint pain, red tongue with yellow fur, and a rapid stringlike pulse. Synonym: "kidney channel malaria."

Wasting-thirst, *xiāo kě*, 消渴

Refers to diabetes. Primarily due to alcohol addiction, indulgence in sweet and fatty foods, spleen and stomach damp–heat; or caused by excessive among the five minds giving rise to depressed fire; or sexual overindulgence giving rise to frenetic stirring of vacuity fire and consumption of kidney essence. Manifesting symptoms include thirst with increased fluid intake, a large intake of food, and copious urine. According to the different signs and symptoms, wasting-thirst disease can be categorized into three groups: wasting-thirst of the upper, center, and lower burners.

PD (p.142): Dispersion-thirst: Synonym: "wasting-thirst." 1. Any disease characterized by thirst, increased fluid intake, and copious urine, and categorized as upper burner, center burner, and lower burner dispersion, depending on the pathomechanism.

Water swelling, *shuǐ zhǒng*, 水腫

PD (p.668): Swelling of the flesh arising when organ dysfunction (spleen, kidney, lung) due to internal or external causes allows water to accumulate. Water swelling stands in contradistinction to toxin swelling, which denotes a localized swelling due to the local presence of toxin as in the case of welling-abscess, flat-abscess, boils, clove sores, and other sores.

Welling-abscess, *yōng*, 癰

PD (p.670):

1. Synonym: "external welling-abscess." A large suppuration in the flesh characterized by a painful swelling and redness that is clearly circumscribed, and that before rupturing is soft and characterized by a thin shiny skin. It may be

associated with generalized heat [effusion], thirst, yellow tongue fur and a rapid pulse.
2. Synonym: "internal welling-abscess." A suppuration in the chest or abdomen affecting the organs; probably so called because it shares many of the *yang* qualities of external welling-abscess, except for its location in the body.

Wind strike, *zhòng fēng*, 中風
PD (p.691): Synonym: "wind stroke." 1. The sudden appearance of hemiplegia, deviated eyes and mouth, and impeded speech that may or may not start with sudden clouding collapse (loss of consciousness). In *The Inner Canon* (*Nèi Jīng*), the term *zhòng fēng* is used in the general sense of contracting wind evil.

Wind–water, *fēng shuǐ*, 風水
PD (p.694): External wind contraction with water swelling. Signs include rapid onset, floating pulse, pain in the joints, heat effusion and aversion to cold, and swelling, particularly of the head and face (the upper part of the body being affected by wind evil). The disease is the result of impairment of lung *qi*'s depurative downbearing by wind evil in patients suffering from spleen-kidney *qi* vacuity.

Yang brightness disease, *yáng míng bìng*, 陽明病
One of the six-channel diseases. A disease primarily caused by exuberant heat damaging the fluids and heat binding in the intestines and stomach. The main symptoms are abdominal pain that refuses pressure, fecal blockage, tidal fever, delirious speech in severe cases, and a sunken, forceful pulse.

PD (p.698): A disease arising when externally contracted evil enters the *yang* brightness channel and exterior signs such as aversion to wind and cold give way to pronounced heat signs. *Yang* brightness disease is characterized by generalized heat [effusion], sweating and aversion to heat, agitation, and thirst, or, in more severe cases, abdominal fullness and pain, constipation, and, in severe cases, delirious mania. The tongue fur is usually dry and old yellow in color. The pulse is generally surging and large, slippery and rapid, or sunken, replete, and forceful.

Yang pattern, *yáng zhèng*, 陽證
Any pattern with characteristics attributable to *yang* is called a *yang* pattern. For example, exterior pattern, heat pattern, and repletion pattern all belong in the category of *yang* patterns.
Common clinical symptoms of *yang* patterns: Red facial complexion, scorching hot skin and flesh, vexation and agitation, constipation, short voidings of

reddish urine, a crimson red tongue with yellow tongue fur, and a pulse that is floating and rapid, or surging and large.

PD (p. 700): 1. Any exterior pattern, heat pattern, or repletion pattern, especially repletion heat characterized by signs such as heat effusion with aversion to cold, red facial complexion, headache, generalized heat [effusion] with a liking for coolness, manic agitation, dry cracked lips, vexation and thirst with taking of fluids, rough strident voice, rough breathing, constipation or foul-smelling stool, abdominal pain that refuses pressure, short voidings of reddish urine, red tongue with dry yellow fur, and a forceful floating, surging, rapid pulse. 2. Of sores, the presentation of signs such as redness, swelling, hardness, and pain.

Yin and *yang* toxin, *yīn yáng dú*, 陰陽毒

Epidemic toxin; refers to infectious, pathogenic evil *qi*. Exposure to this can lead to the spread of epidemic disease.

Epidemic toxin can be classified as *yang* toxin or *yin* toxin. *Yang* toxin is caused by heat evil congestion and stagnation in the upper body, the main symptoms of which are a red face with brocade-like macules, sore throat, and vomiting of pus and blood. *Yin* toxin is *yin* evil causing obstruction and stagnation in the channels, the main symptoms of which are a blue-green facial complexion and eyes, generalized body pain (as if due to physical injury), and sore throat.

Yin humor, *yīn yè*, 陰毒

PD (p. 710): Essence, blood, liquid, and humor, viewed as *yin*-natured entities in contrast to *yang qi*.

Yin pattern, *yīn zhèng*, 陰證

Any pattern with characteristics attributable to *yin* is called a *yin* pattern. For example, interior pattern, cold pattern, and vacuity pattern all belong to the category of *yin* patterns.

Common clinical symptoms of *yin* patterns: A pale white facial complexion, listlessness of essence-spirit, physical cold and cold limbs, fatigue and lack of strength, a low voice, a bland taste in the mouth, absence of thirst, long voidings of clear urine, a pale red tongue with white tongue fur, and a pulse that is sunken and slow, or fine and rough.

PD (p. 711): 1. Any interior, cold, or vacuity pattern, e.g., somber white or dark dull complexion, curled-up lying posture, cold limbs, inactivity and tendency to talk little, low faint voice, faint weak breathing, shortness of breath and lack of strength, reduced food intake, bland taste in the mouth, absence of vexation and thirst or desire for warm drinks, sloppy stool, long voidings of clear urine, abdominal pain that likes pressure, pale enlarged tongue, glossy slimy tongue fur, and a forceless sunken slow fine pulse. 2. A pattern in which sores of any kind present with broad roots, with paleness of the skin in the affected area, and with absence of heat, swelling, redness, and pain.

■ Herbal Formulas

Aconite Main Tuber Decoction, *Wū Tóu Tāng*, 烏頭湯
Ingredients: *Zhì chuān wū* (Aconiti Radix preparata), *má huáng* (Ephedrae Herba), *bái sháo* (Paeoniae Radix alba), *huáng qí* (Astragali Radix), and *zhì gān cǎo* (Glycyrrhizae Radix preparata).
Actions: Warms the channels, courses wind, and relieves pain.

Astragalus and Cinnamon Twig Five Agents Decoction,
***Huáng Qí Guì Zhī Wǔ Wù Tāng*, 黃耆桂枝五物湯**
Ingredients: *Huáng qí* (Astragali Radix), *sháo yào* (Paeoniae Radix alba; Paeoniae Radix rubra), *guì zhī* (Cinnamomi Ramulus), *shēng jiāng* (Zingiberis Rhizoma recens), and *dà zǎo* (Jujubae Fructus).
Actions: Boosts the qi, warms and harmonizes the channels, and frees impediment.

Atractylodes and Aconite Decoction, *Bái Zhú Fù Zǐ Tāng*, 白术附子湯
Ingredients: *Páo fù zǐ* (Aconiti Radix lateralis preparata, blast-fried), *bái zhú* (Atractylodis macrocephalae Rhizoma), *shēng jiāng* (Zingiberis Rhizoma recens), *zhì gān cǎo* (Glycyrrhizae Radix preparata), and *dà zǎo* (Jujubae Fructus).
Actions: Warms the channels and dissipates cold; fortifies the spleen and eliminates dampness.

Cimicifuga Decoction, *Shēng Má Tāng*, 升麻湯
Ingredients: *Shēng má* (Cimicifugae Rhizoma), *fú shén* (Poriae Sclerotium pararadicis), *rén shēn* (Ginseng Radix), *fáng fēng* (Saposhnikoviae Radix), *xī jiǎo* (Rhinocerotis Cornu), *líng yáng jiǎo* (Saigae tataricae Cornu), *qiāng huó* (Notopterygii Rhizoma seu Radix), and *guì zhī* (Cinnamomi Ramulus).*

Cinnamon Twig and Aconite Decoction, *Guì Zhī Fù Zǐ Tāng*, 桂枝附子湯
Ingredients: *Guī zhī* (Cinnamomi Ramulus), *bái sháo* (Paeoniae Radix alba), *shēng jiāng* (Zingiberis Rhizoma recens), *dà zǎo* (Jujubae Fructus), *gān cǎo* (Glycyrrhizae Radix), and *fù zǐ* (Aconiti Radix lateralis preparata).

---

* Since most countries have laws ban the trade of any parts of endangered animals, the use of *xī jiǎo* (rhinoceros horn) and *líng yáng jiǎo* (antelope horn) is now forbidden in some countries. For more information, see CITES treaty (the Convention on International Trade in Endangered Species of Wild Fauna and Flora).

Cinnamon Twig Decoction Plus Astragalus Decoction, *Guì Zhī Jiā Huáng Qí Tāng,* 桂枝加黃耆湯

Ingredients: *Guī zhī* (Cinnamomi Ramulus), *sháo yào* (Paeoniae Radix alba; Paeoniae Radix rubra), *gān cǎo* (Glycyrrhizae Radix), *shēng jiāng* (Zingiberis Rhizoma recens), *dà zǎo* (Jujubae Fructus), and *huáng qí* (Astragali Radix).

Actions: Harmonizes construction (*yíng,* 營) and defense (*wèi,* 衛); frees constrained *yang.*

Cinnamon Twig Decoction Plus Dragon Bone and Oyster Shell, *Guī Zhī Jiā Lóng Gǔ Mǔ Lì Tang,* 桂枝加龍骨牡蠣湯

Ingredients: *Guī zhī* (Cinnamomi Ramulus), *bái sháo* (Paeoniae Radix alba), *lóng gǔ* (Fossilia Ossis Mastodi), *mǔ lì* (Ostreae Concha), *shēng jiāng* (Zingiberis Rhizoma recens), *dà zǎo* (Jujubae Fructus), and *gān cǎo* (Glycyrrhizae Radix).

Actions: Constrains the essence, suppresses counterflow, and regulates and harmonizes the *yin* and *yang.*

Cinnamon Twig, Peony, and Anemarrhena Decoction, *Guī Zhī Sháo Yào Zhī Mǔ Tāng,* 桂枝芍藥知母湯

Ingredients: *Guī zhī* (Cinnamomi Ramulus), *má huáng* (Ephedrae Herba), *fù zǐ* (Aconiti Radix lateralis preparata), *zhī mǔ* (Anemarrhenae Rhizoma), *sháo yào* (Paeoniae Radix alba; Paeoniae Radix rubra), *bái zhú* (Atractylodis macrocephalae Rhizoma), *fáng fēng* (Saposhnikoviae Radix), *shēng jiāng* (Zingiberis Rhizoma recens), and *gān cǎo* (Glycyrrhizae Radix).

Actions: Frees the flow of *yang qi,* promotes movement (in areas with impediment), dispels wind, and vanquishes dampness.

Dichroa Leaf Powder, *Shǔ Qī Sǎn,* 蜀漆散

Ingredients: *Shǔ qī* (Dichroae Folium), *yún mǔ* (Muscovitum), and *lóng gǔ* (Fossilia Ossis Mastodi).

Actions: Dispels phlegm and interrupts illness.

Ephedra Decoction, *Má Huáng Tāng,* 麻黃湯

Ingredients: *Má huáng* (Ephedrae Herba), *guì zhī* (Cinnamomi Ramulus), *xìng rén* (Armeniacae Semen amarum), *zhì gān cǎo* (Glycyrrhizae Radix preparata).

Actions: Resolves exterior cold and suppresses panting.

Fangji Decoction, *Fáng Jǐ Tāng,* 防己湯

Ingredients: *Fáng jǐ* (Stephaniae Radix), *fú líng* (Poria), *bái zhú* (Atractylodis macrocephalae Rhizoma), *guì xīn* (Cinnamomi Cortex), *shēng jiāng* (Zingiberis

Rhizoma recens), *wū tóu* (Aconiti Radix), *rén shēn* (Ginseng Radix), and *gān cǎo* (Glycyrrhizae Radix).

Flavescent Sophora Decoction, *Kǔ Shēn Tāng*, 苦參湯
Ingredients: *Kǔ shēn* (Sophorae flavescentis Radix), *dì yú* (Sanguisorbae Radix), *huáng lián* (Coptidis Rhizoma), *wáng bù liú xíng* (Vaccariae Semen), *dú huó* (Angelicae pubescentis Radix), *ài yè* (Artemisiae argyi Folium), and *zhú yè* (Lophateri Herba).

Heart-Draining Decoction, *Xiè Xīn Tāng*, 瀉心湯
Ingredients: *Dà huáng* (Rhei Radix et Rhizoma), *huáng lián* (Coptidis Rhizoma), and *huáng qín* (Scutellariae Radix).
Actions: Drains fire, resolves toxin, and dries dampness.

Kidney *Qi* Pill, *Shèn Qì Wán*, 腎氣丸
Ingredients: *Gān dì huáng* (Rehmanniae Radix recens), *shǔ yù [shān yào]* (Dioscoreae Rhizoma), *shān zhū yú* (Corni Fructus), *zé xiè* (Alismatis Rhizoma), *fú líng* (Poria), *mǔ dān pí* (Moutan Cortex), *guì zhī* (Cinnamomi Ramulus), and *páo fù zǐ* (Aconiti Radix lateralis preparata, blast-fried).
Actions: Warms and supplements kidney *yang*.

Licorice Decoction, *Gān Cǎo Tāng*, 甘草湯
Ingredients: *Shēng gān cǎo* (Glycyrrhizae Radix).
Actions: Clears heat and resolves toxin; disinhibits the throat and relieves pain.

Major Aconite Main Tuber Decoction, *Dà Wū Tóu Tāng*, 大烏頭湯
(*The Pulse Classic*: same as Aconite Main Tuber Decoction, *Wū Tóu Tāng*, 大烏頭湯)

Major *Qi*-Coordinating Decoction, *Dà Chéng Qì Tāng*, 大承氣湯
Ingredients: *Dà huáng* (Rhei Radix et Rhizoma) [add near end], *máng xiāo* (Natrii Sulfas) [dissolve in strained decoction], *zhǐ shí* (Aurantii Fructus immaturus), and *hòu pò* (Magnoliae officinalis Cortex).
Actions: Vigorously purges heat accumulation.

Minor Center-Fortifying Decoction, *Xiao Jiàn Zhōng Tāng*, 小建中湯
Ingredients: *Sháo yào* (Paeoniae Radix alba; Paeoniae Radix rubra), *guì zhī* (Cinnamomi Ramulus), *shēng jiāng* (Zingiberis Rhizoma recens), *dà zǎo* (Jujubae Fructus), *zhì gān cǎo* (Glycyrrhizae Radix preparata), and *yí táng* (Maltosum).

Actions: Warms and supplements the center burner and moderates spasmodic abdominal pain.

Minor Pinellia Decoction, *Xiǎo Bàn Xià Tāng,* 小半夏湯
Ingredients: *Bàn xià* (Pinelliae Rhizoma), *zhú rú* (Bambusae Caulis in taeniam), *rén shēn* (Ginseng Radix), *gān cǎo* (Glycyrrhizae Radix), *shēng jiāng* (Zingiberis Rhizoma recens), and *dà zǎo* (Jujubae Fructus).
Actions: Boosts *qi* and downbears counterflow; rectifies *qi* and transforms phlegm.

Niter and Alum Powder, *Xiāo Shí Fán Shí Sǎn,* 硝石礜石散
Ingredients: *Xiāo shí* (Nitrum) and *fán shí* (Alum).

Officinal Magnolia Bark Seven Agents Decoction, *Hòu Pò Qī Wù Tāng,* 厚朴七物湯
Ingredients: *Hòu pò* (Magnoliae officinalis Cortex), *gān cǎo* (Glycyrrhizae Radix), *dà huáng* (Rhei Radix et Rhizoma), *zhǐ shí* (Aurantii Fructus immaturus), *guì zhī* (Cinnamomi Ramulus), *shēng jiāng* (Zingiberis Rhizoma recens), and *dà zǎo* (Jujubae Fructus).
Actions: Resolves the flesh and the exterior, promotes the movement of *qi*, and frees the stool.

Officinal Magnolia Bark Three Agents Decoction, *Hòu Pò Sān Wù Tāng,* 厚朴三物湯
Ingredients: *Hòu pò* (Magnoliae officinalis Cortex), *zhǐ shí* (Aurantii Fructus immaturus), and *dà huáng* (Rhei Radix et Rhizoma).
Actions: Drains *qi* downward and frees the stool.

Pueraria Decoction, *Gé Gēn Tāng,* 葛根湯
Ingredients: *Gé gēn* (Puerariae Radix), *má huáng* (Ephedrae Herba), *guì zhī* (Cinnamomi Ramulus), *sháo yào* (Paeoniae Radix alba; Paeoniae Radix rubra), *shēng jiāng* (Zingiberis Rhizoma recens), *dà zǎo* (Jujubae Fructus), and *gān cǎo* (Glycyrrhizae Radix).
Actions: Resolves the exterior and the flesh, and engenders fluids.

Rhubarb and Aconite Decoction, *Dà Huáng Fù Zǐ Tāng,* 大黃附子湯
Ingredients: *Fù zǐ* (Aconiti Radix lateralis preparata), *dà huáng* (Rhei Radix et Rhizoma), and *xì xīn* (Asari Herba).
Actions: Warms the interior, disperses cold, frees the stool, and relieves pain.

Rhubarb, Phellodendron, Gardenia, and Mirabilitum Decoction,
Dà Huáng Huáng Bǎi Zhī Zǐ Máng Xiāo Tāng, 大黃黃柏梔子芒硝湯
Ingredients: *Dà huáng* (Rhei Radix et Rhizoma), *huáng bǎi* (Phellodendri Cortex), *zhī zǐ* (Gardeniae Fructus), and *máng xiāo* (Natrii Sulfas).

Rice Bean and Chinese Angelica Decoction, Chì Xiǎo Dòu Dāng Guī Tāng,
赤小豆當歸湯
Ingredients: *Chì xiǎo dòu* (Phaseoli Semen), *dāng guī* (Angelicae sinensis Radix), and *jiàng shuǐ* (sour millet water [Setariae Praeparatum Liquidum]).
Actions: Percolates dampness and clears heat; resolves toxin and transforms stasis; expels pus.

Running Piglet Decoction, Bēn Tún Tāng, 奔豚湯
Ingredients: *Gān cǎo* (Glycyrrhizae Radix), *chuān xiōng* (Chuanxiong Rhizoma), *dāng guī* (Angelicae sinensis Radix), *bàn xià* (Piubelliae Rhizoma), *huáng qín* (Scutellariae Radix), *shēng gé* (Puerariae Radicis Recentis), *sháo yào* (Paeoniae Radix alba; Paeoniae Radix rubra), *shēng jiāng* (Zingiberis Rhizoma recens), and *gān lǐ gēn bái pí* (Pruni Salicinae Radicis Cortex).
Actions: Dispels cold, downbears counterflow *qi*, warms the *yang*, and regulates the *qi*.

Trichosanthes, Chinese Chive, and White Liquor Decoction,
Guā Lóu Xiè Bái Bái Jiǔ Tāng, 栝蔞薤白白酒湯
Ingredients: *Guā lóu* (Trichosanthis Fructus), *xiè bái* (Allii macrostemi Bulbus), and *bái jiǔ* (Chinese white liquor [Granorum Spiritus Incolor]).
Actions: Frees the *yang*, promotes the movement of *qi*, and expels phlegm.

Trichosanthes and Cinnamon Twig Decoction, Guā Lóu Guì Zhī Tāng,
栝蔞桂枝湯
Ingredients: *Guā lóu gēn* (Trichosanthis Radix), *guì zhī* (Cinnamomi Ramulus), *sháo yào* (Paeoniae Radix alba; Paeoniae Radix rubra), *zhì gān cǎo* (Glycyrrhizae Radix preparata), *shēng jiāng* (Zingiberis Rhizoma recens), and *dà zǎo* (Jujubae Fructus).
Actions: Soothes the sinews and channels; engenders fluids.

Turtle Shell Decocted Pill, Biē Jiǎ Jiān Wán, 鱉甲煎丸
Ingredients: *Biē jiǎ* (Trionycis Carapax), *wū shàn [shè gān]* (Belamcandae Rhizoma), *huáng qín* (Scutellariae Radix), *shǔ fù* (Armadillidium), *chái hú* (Bupleuri Radix), *tíng lì zǐ* (Lepidii/Descurainiae Semen), *shí wéi* (Pyrrosiae Folium), *hòu pò* (Magnoliae officinalis Cortex), *dān pí* (Moutan Cortex), *qú mài* (Dianthi Herba),

zǐ wēi (Campsitis Grandiflorae Flos), *bàn xià* (Pinelliae Rhizoma), *rén shēn* (Ginseng Radix), *zhé chóng* (Eupolyphaga seu Steleophaga), *ē jiāo* (Asini Corii Colla), *fēng fáng* (Vespae Nidus), *chì xiāo* (Nitrum Rubrum), *qiāng láng* (Catharsius), and *táo rén* (Persicae Semen).

Actions: Breaks blood and expels stasis; softens hardness and dissipates binds; supplements vacuity and regulates construction (*yíng*, 營).

White Chicken's Dropping Powder, *Jī Shǐ Bái Sǎn*, 雞屎白散
Ingredients: *Jī shǐ bái* (Galli Faeces Albae).

White Tiger Decoction, *Bái Hǔ Tāng*, 白虎湯
Ingredients: *Shí gāo* (Gypsum fibrosum), *zhī mǔ* (Anemarrhenae Rhizoma), *zhì gān cǎo* (Glycyrrhizae Radix preparata), and *jīng mǐ* (Oryza sativa L.).
Actions: Clears heat in the *qi* aspect, drains stomach fire, engenders fluids, and relieves thirst.

White Tiger Decoction Plus Cinnamon Twig Decoction, *Bái Hǔ Jiā Guì Zhī Tāng*, 白虎加桂枝湯
Ingredients: *Shí gāo* (Gypsum fibrosum), *zhī mǔ* (Anemarrhenae Rhizoma), *gān cǎo* (Glycyrrhizae Radix), *jīng mǐ* (Oryza sativa L.), and *guī zhī* (Cinnamomi Ramulus).
Actions: Clears heat, boosts *qi*, and engenders fluid.

■ Index